D0394380

ADDITIONAL PRAISE FOR *5 POUNDS*

"Harley Pasternak's *5 Pounds* is a clearly written, practical approach to both full-body fat loss and overall wellness. Based on data from scientific studies, Harley provides easy to follow, step-by-step instructions designed to jumpstart a fat loss/wellness program. For those who have struggled with losing body fat or keeping it off, I highly recommend trying this program."
—**Peter Lemon, PhD, FACSM,**
professor and Weider Research Chair
at Western University

"Harley knows the secrets to achieving a killer physique and making the workouts fun: I've never been in better shape and I feel amazing! He is a genius."
—**Behati Prinsloo,**
Victoria's Secret angel, supermodel

"Harley has a gift for translating complex and important exercise and nutrition research into a program that's easy to implement."
—**Ira Jacobs, DrMedSc,**
Dean, faculty of Kinesiology & Physical Education
at the University of Toronto

"The best part about working with Harley is that he is constantly evolving and giving his clients the most current, cutting-edge research. His latest 5-day plan is so doable, effective, and straightforward that it is difficult not to follow!"
—**Jordana Brewster,**
actress

**Lose the First,
Lose the Last,
LOSE IT FAST!**

5

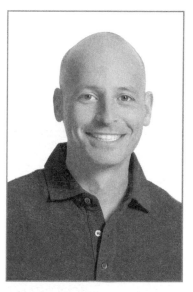

POUNDS

THE BREAKTHROUGH 5-DAY PLAN to JUMP-START RAPID WEIGHT LOSS (AND NEVER GAIN IT BACK!)

HARLEY PASTERNAK, MSc

NEW YORK TIMES BESTSELLING AUTHOR

For Jess and Liv

Internet addresses and telephone numbers given in this book
were accurate at the time it went to press.

© 2015 by Harley Pasternak

All rights reserved. No part of this publication may be reproduced or transmitted in any form or by any means, electronic or mechanical, including photocopying, recording, or any other information storage and retrieval system, without the written permission of the publisher.

Rodale books may be purchased for business or promotional use or for special sales. For information, please write to: Special Markets Department, Rodale, Inc., 733 Third Avenue, New York, NY 10017

Printed in the United States of America

Rodale Inc. makes every effort to use acid-free ♾, recycled paper ♻.

Photographs by Beth Bischoff

Book design by Elizabeth Neal and Amy King

Library of Congress Cataloging-in-Publication Data is on file with the publisher.

ISBN-13: 978–1–62336–457–1

Distributed to the trade by Macmillan

2   4   6   8   10   9   7   5   3   1   hardcover

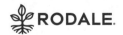

We inspire and enable people to improve their lives and the world around them.
rodalebooks.com

CONTENTS

Acknowledgments   vi

Introduction   vii

PART 1:
The My 5 Plan   1

Chapter 1: **(PROTEIN + FIBER) X 5**   2

Chapter 2: **FLEX YOUR MUSCLES DAILY**   25

Chapter 3: **WALK IT OFF**   49

Chapter 4: **SNOOZE TO LOSE**   75

Chapter 5: **PULL THE CORD**   98

PART 2:
5 Days 5 Pounds   119

Chapter 6: **THE 5-DAY DIET**   120

Chapter 7: **SAY YES TO SUCCESS**   131

Chapter 8: **MY 5 FOR LIFE**   144

Chapter 9: **WHY YOU'LL NEVER REGAIN THE POUNDS**   160

PART 3:
Recipes   173

PART 4:
The My 5 Workouts   215

GET STARTED   216

ADD VARIETY   224

TAKE IT UP A NOTCH   232

PART 5:
Journal Pages   243

Notes   258

Index   287

ACKNOWLEDGMENTS

I'd like to thank the following people for helping make this book a reality:

Olivia Bell Buehl for turning my ideas into clear and coherent sentences.

Allison Garfield for making the perfect edits.

Corinne Babiolakis and Arash Bandegan for compiling an almost endless amount of research.

Andrea Barzvi of Empire Literary. Here's to our sixth book together.

Ursula Cary, Yelena Nesbit, Amy King, and the rest of the team at Rodale for such a great partnership.

Beth Bischoff for the great photography.

Susan Lilly Ott for the yummy (and easy) recipes.

My clients for following most of my advice and being great guinea pigs.

My partners Tim Rosa for counting my steps, Tara Piper for keeping me hydrated, Caitlin Wholey for keeping my feet comfortable and fly, and Cory Saenz for the protein.

INTRODUCTION

You've lost weight before. Maybe even several times. But you're still not happy with your body. Perhaps, despite all your efforts, you're heavier than ever. Or maybe it's that you just can't shake those last few pounds. You care about how you look. You know what you're "supposed" to eat. You belong to a gym.

So why can't you drop the pounds and get the body you want—and deserve—especially given all your hard work?

After a decade of studying weight loss as an undergrad and a graduate student at university, then 3 years as a scientist, and nearly 22 years in private practice, even I've become confused, overwhelmed, and often immobilized by all the weight-loss information we're bombarded with. Every morning I wake up to a new slew of studies, all announcing yet another "thing" that can help us lose weight, burn calories, and banish fat.

Putting aside all those silly methods marketed to us in books and magazines, on television and the Internet—think of the Cookie Diet, the Caveman Diet, fat-burning cleanses, pole-dancing workouts, etc.—there are countless actions supported by good science that can help you slim down. Examples: drinking cold water or green tea, eating more loganberries and grapefruit and whole grains, laughing and fidgeting more, exercising in cold weather, replacing your desk chair with a stability ball, getting a workout partner, keeping a diet log, and so on, and on, and on.

In fact, there are so many things we can do, eat, use, or avoid to help us lose weight that we could spend every minute of our days trying to execute even a small fraction of the items on that list. And forget about your commitments to your job and your family. And oh, yeah, how about sleep?

So which of these things do we actually need to do? Which ones make the most difference? And which take the least amount of time? Bottom line: Which are the absolutely most effective and efficient behaviors we need to incorporate into our lives to lose the most amount of weight in the least amount of time? And while we're at it, how can we do so without having to buy special food, expensive supplements, fancy exercise equipment, or a gym membership?

In search of the Holy Grail of weight loss, I recruited scientists at three of the top North American universities, and together we examined the vast body of weight-loss research recorded over the past few decades to see which weight-loss habits proved to be the most effective. Then, I reviewed two decades' worth of client notes and logs from my own practice as a nutritionist and fitness trainer. Finally, after narrowing down that list, I tried out those behaviors, first on myself, and then on my clients.

Two years later, I have the answer. I've distilled the essence of weight loss into five simple actions that complement one another and work synergistically. All will make you look and feel your best . . . today . . . this week . . . forever.

That means you'll no longer have to waste your time, money, and energy experimenting with what *might* work, only to see no (or minimal) results. I've done the work and figured it out for you.

This book introduces a revolutionary plan to slim down. It's revolutionary because it's so *easy*. Anyone can do it. All you have to do is follow five easy steps for 5 days and you'll lose 5 pounds. And that's a promise! It's also revolutionary because the results you'll achieve during those 5 days will transform the way you eat, sleep, exercise, and more—for good. I call it the "My 5 Plan" because it reflects my synergistic approach to weight loss, and it will soon become your blueprint for the best body you've ever had.

For many of you, dropping 5 pounds in 5 days will be just the beginning of your journey. With that immediate success under your (newly tightened) belt, you'll be motivated to keep going, to watch more pounds melt away until you reach your ideal weight. And all it requires is continuing to follow the simple My 5 Plan—which won't even feel like a plan after long. It's actually a healthy lifestyle for a brand-new you.

After all, as anyone who has experienced the yo-yo effect of losing weight on a diet program only to soon regain it (and often a few extra pounds for good measure) knows, you have to stick with the program to maintain your weight loss. The big difference with My 5 is that it doesn't feel like a diet. It's so easy to do and delivers such noticeable, immediate results that there's absolutely no need to revert to your old way of eating. I'll also give you plenty of advice on how to maintain your new (or evolving) shape in the months and years to come. As you incorporate these small but powerful changes into your lifestyle, you'll finally take control of your weight, once and for all.

My 5 won't add to your already busy schedule, other than the need to do about 5 minutes of resistance exercise each day. I'll take you step by step through these resistance exercises with photos and instructions. And by the way, not to worry, I designed the exercises to be adaptable to your fitness level—even if lying on the couch is currently your most strenuous activity! You're already doing three of the other pieces of the program: eating, moving, and sleeping. You'll also pick up an hour a day when you detach yourself from your electronic devices—that's the surprising but highly effective fifth component.

In the following chapters, you'll learn everything you need to know to change your body, your metabolism, and your sense of control over your weight. You'll be amazed at how simple the program is. You'll come to understand the hows and whys of each behavior and the ways they complement one another. Plus, I'll give you lots of practical tips on how to get meals on the table fast, using a minimum of ingredients.

At the end of each day, you'll answer five simple questions. If you can respond with a resounding *yes* to each, you'll be 5 pounds lighter at the end of Day 5.

As ancient Greek philosopher Aristotle famously noted, "The whole is greater than the sum of its parts." And of course the German language has given us a word for something that's made from many parts but is somehow more than or different from their total: *gestalt.* My 5 includes five changes in behavior, and when you engage in all of them, the synergistic effect is much greater. And your reward will be subtracting a minimum of 5 pounds, which might well translate into a smaller dress or pants size. You'll also be amazed at how much better you feel.

With only 5 days to achieve these results, let's not waste another minute. It's time to get going!

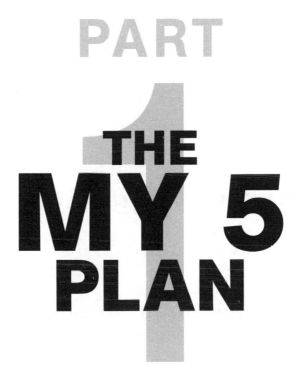

PART

1

THE
MY 5
PLAN

CHAPTER 1

(PROTEIN + FIBER) X

Changing the way you eat is obviously essential to weight loss. But that alone is unlikely to result in the kind of weight loss you're looking for. It's only one of the five interlocking factors that make up my revolutionary approach to fast-track weight loss. After 22 years of working one-on-one to help people lose weight, I have a pretty good handle on human nature. If I begin with any of the other four components, I know that you will likely skip over the other content to see what you can eat, when you can eat it, and how much of it you can eat. So I'll save you the trouble. However, I want to reiterate that following just the dietary prescription and ignoring the rest of My 5, or choosing only the components you like best, will not give you the results promised in the title: goodbye to 5 pounds— fast! The My 5 eating plan "formula" for success isn't just fast. It's also simple: Eat three meals and two snacks that include protein and fiber each and every day.

Five Reasons Why My 5 Is Easy to Do

1. You don't have to count calories.

2. You don't have to weigh portions.

3. You'll find the foods you need in any well-stocked supermarket, so there's no need to seek out exotic ingredients or to order expensive special meals.

4. You won't be overcome by cravings or extreme hunger.

5. You can easily eat this way anywhere: at home, at work, and on the road.

WHAT, WHEN, AND HOW MUCH?

The food component of My 5 has three aspects:

1. *Frequency:* You'll eat five times a day (three meals and two snacks).

2. *Food choices:* Every meal must have protein, fibrous carbohydrates—think leafy greens, string beans, apples, and lots more—and healthy fats. Snacks, too, must contain protein and fibrous carbs.

3. *Portion control:* You'll use your hand to judge portion size.

Follow all three guidelines for optimal results. (That's a polite way of saying no straying!) I'll go into greater detail about each of these factors in the pages that follow and provide you with a week's worth of detailed meal plans, starting on page 126.

EAT FIVE TIMES A DAY

Two of my professors at the University of Toronto, David Jenkins, MD, PhD, and Thomas M.S. Wolever, MD, PhD, pioneered the research that laid out the case for eating several small meals rather than three large ones, which underlies this program.[1] The pair also created the glycemic index. (See "A Glimpse at the Glycemic Index" on page 19.)

Eating three meals and two snacks spaced out evenly throughout the day is not optional; it's absolutely integral to My 5. You'll be eating roughly every 3 hours. Say you have breakfast at 7:00 a.m. Then you'd have your morning snack at 10:00 a.m., followed by lunch at 1:00 p.m. At 4:00 p.m., you'd have another snack, followed by dinner at 7:00 p.m. Obviously, you can adjust these times to fit your schedule, but the point is to never allow yourself to become overly hungry by going more than 4 hours between a meal or a snack.

Why does this approach work so well? I'm sure you've had the experience of postponing lunch or dinner for hours, only to find that when you did sit down to eat, you were insatiable. You grabbed the first thing you saw and as much of it as you could—think potato chips, candy, or baked goods. That's *reactive* eating. Instead, I want you to eat *proactively,* which enables you to remain in control of your appetite and what and how much you eat. And obviously, appetite control is a key component of weight loss. But the neat thing is that you're not *suppressing* your appetite to control your intake. Instead, your appetite is actually reduced when you eat more frequently, and your cravings also disappear. That's why I refer to this concept as "grazing rather than gorging."

Why does eating this way help you lose weight? There's been considerable research comparing the impact of eating more, smaller meals each day (grazing) with the conventional three-meals-a-day approach. Studies show that the grazing method helps moderate blood sugar levels, resulting in lower insulin levels, which is essential to weight loss.[2, 3] Grazing also reduces appetite[4-9] and minimizes cravings for sweet and starchy foods. Other studies suggest that eating frequent meals leads to a steadier metabolism, which can burn more fat throughout the day[10, 11] as well as give you a more consistent energy level throughout the day.[12, 13] Because less body fat is stored, rapid weight loss can result and can be maintained.[15, 16] Finally, in concert with eating sufficient protein, grazing rather than gorging enhances the ability to maintain muscle mass while losing weight.[17-19]

Five Benefits of Grazing

1. Better control of blood sugar and insulin levels.

2. A more consistent metabolism and energy level throughout the day.

3. The lack of extreme hunger and cravings for sweet or starchy foods.

4. Rapid weight loss because less fat is stored.

5. The ability to maintain lean muscle mass while losing weight.

NO CALORIE COUNTING

Awareness of calories is important to portion control, but you won't actually have to count them on the My 5 Plan as long as you follow the meal plan guidelines and use your hand to gauge portion sizes. (You'll learn how in Chapter 6.) However, if *not* counting calories makes you nervous, you'll be reassured to know that each day you'll consume roughly 1,300 to 1,400 calories if you currently weigh less than 175 pounds and 1,600 to 1,700 calories if you currently weigh 175 pounds or more. That breaks down to 350 to 450 calories a meal, again, depending on your size, and about 150 calories per snack. These calorie levels facilitate expedited weight loss, in concert with regular activity.[20]

While I'm on the subject of calories, let me add that the overwhelming focus on calories has sidetracked nutritionists, physicians, and the food industry for more than half a century. (I could say the same for carbohydrates.) What matters most is the nutritional value of foods. I'm not saying we should *ignore* calories—eating too much of any food will pack on the pounds. But the focus on calories has obscured the fact that equally important is that different types of foods and when we eat them affect our hormones and even our brain messaging.[21, 22]

Protein calories don't behave in your body the same way that fat or carb calories do.[23-25] In fact, a high-protein diet can burn up to 100 extra calories a day without any additional activity. Certain foods are more satiating, meaning they're more filling, namely those with high levels of fat, protein, and/or fiber. Eating 200 calories of eggs will make you feel fuller or feel fuller sooner than eating the same number of calories of a donut.[26] So, once and for all, calories are important, but they are only one piece of the puzzle inherent in achieving weight loss.

MEET THE MACRONUTRIENTS

The three major macronutrients (food groups) we build a diet around are protein, carbohydrate, and fat. We cannot thrive for very long without one or more of these food groups. Each one is essential to our health and contributes to organ function, energy, cell repair, hormone creation, and a host of other effects, all the way down to creating healthy hair and nails. The relative amounts of these three macronutrients in your meals play a role in weight loss, as does their quality.

While some foods are exclusively or almost exclusively one category of macronutrient (egg white is protein, olive oil is fat, grapes are carbohydrate), most are a combination of two or three macronutrients. For example, chicken is part protein and part fat, while milk and lentils and other beans contain carbohydrate, fat, and protein. The meals and snacks you'll be eating on the My 5 Plan contain all three macronutrients in a certain balance. Let's look briefly at each macronutrient before discussing how they'll come together in your meals and snacks and work in concert to help you lose weight.

THE PROTEIN PACKAGE

Think of protein as a train with many adjoining cars, and each train car as one amino acid. Most of our body mass that isn't water is made up of protein, including our organs, muscles, and skin. Protein contains 4 calories per gram, and because our body cannot store protein (as it does fat and carbohydrate), higher protein consumption doesn't easily translate to gaining body fat. Any excess the body doesn't use is simply excreted. (In some extreme cases, protein can be converted to carbohydrate, which can be then converted into fat.) In other words, most people don't gain weight by overeating fish, chicken breast, eggs, or Greek yogurt. With My 5, you'll be eating protein at every meal and snack, and overall getting 30 percent of your calories from protein.

Research on moderately high protein intake provides all sorts of good news to anyone concerned about his or her weight:

- Eating protein (and less carbohydrate) at each meal results in more weight loss than not eating protein throughout the day.[27-30]

- Eating protein at every meal helps preserve muscle mass even as fat is lost.[31]

- Eating adequate protein protects lean muscle mass.[32-35]

- Eating sufficient protein increases fat loss, improving body mass index (BMI).[36, 37]

- Eating protein specifically at breakfast reduces food cravings and intake throughout the rest of the day.[38]

- Eating plenty of protein aids satiety (the opposite of hunger), making it less likely you'll overeat.[39]

Four Reasons to Eat Protein

Here's how protein-rich meals help you slim down fast:

1. They contribute to satiety, so you can eat less and still feel full.

2. They raise your metabolism so you burn more calories.

3. They build and protect (fat-burning) muscle mass.

4. Unlike high-carb meals or snacks, they don't create high insulin levels.

Bottom line: If there's no protein on your plate, it isn't a meal!

PROTEIN ON THE MENU

You'll be eating quality sources of protein on the My 5 Plan:

- Seafood
- Poultry (chicken and turkey)
- Nonfat and low-fat organic dairy
- Beef, pork, and game
- Eggs and egg whites
- Legumes and beans
- Protein powder

PROTEIN FROM THE SEA

Fish and shellfish are wonderful protein sources, as well as great sources of healthy fats, particularly fatty coldwater fish rich in valuable omega-3 and omega-6 fats. It's a good idea to focus on the smaller species that are low on the food chain. They're less likely to contain dangerous levels of mercury. Consume large species only once a week, but not if you're pregnant or breast-feeding. (See "Seafood Selections" below. Also visit the Environmental Defense Fund's Seafood Selector at edf.org/seafood.)

Seafood Selections

COLDWATER FISH	SHELLFISH	OTHER OPTIONS	LARGE SPECIES TO AVOID
Anchovies	Crawfish	Catfish	Halibut
Artic char	King crab	Flounder	King mackerel
Atlantic mackerel	Oysters	Sand dabs	Marlin
Herring	Scallops	Sea bass	Shark
Sardines	Shrimp	Sole	Swordfish
Striped bass		Sturgeon	Tilefish
Trout		Tilapia	Tuna
Wild Alaska salmon			
Wild Pacific salmon			

POULTRY PROTEIN

Chicken and turkey are wonderfully versatile sources of protein that can be grilled, stir-fried, or baked. A few pointers:

- Lean toward white (breast) meat, which receives more of its calories from protein than dark (thigh and leg) meat.

- Purchase skinned breasts or remove the skin before eating.

- Ground lean turkey or chicken breast makes great burgers.

- Turkey jerky is a convenient snack to have on hand.

- Avoid breaded or deep-fried prepared poultry dishes.

THE LOWDOWN ON DAIRY

Did you know that five of the 10 countries with the longest average life span have a diet very high in dairy products? In case you're curious, they're Sweden, France, Italy, Israel, and Greece. Follow these guidelines when purchasing dairy products:

- Use reduced or low-fat products, which are higher in protein and lower in calories.

- Although organic dairy products are more expensive, it's a good idea to use them. The United States is one of the few countries that still allows farmers to inject rBGH (synthetic bovine growth hormone) into cows. A Canadian study indicates that milk from rBGH-treated cows contains significantly elevated levels of insulin-like growth factor I (IGF-I) and presents human health safety concerns.[40] There's also some evidence that a higher milk intake is linked to girls beginning to menstruate early.[41] Organic dairy products contain no rBGH.

- If dairy products give you gas or stomach distress—to a large extent, your ethnic heritage influences how well you can digest milk—use lactose-free products. Greek yogurt, goat milk yogurt, and some low-fat cheeses are also essentially lactose-free.

All Yogurt Is Not Created Equal

Is yogurt a sweet treat filled with fruit and sugar? Or is it a tangy, protein-rich condiment? It's both, of course, but there's a world of difference between regular flavored yogurt and unflavored Greek yogurt, which has been strained to make it thicker. Among the many brands of Greek yogurt in your supermarket are Oikos, Chobani, Fage, and Stonyfield. The chart below compares the nutritional information on the label of a brand of low-fat conventional yogurt with that of a nonfat Greek-style yogurt. Note the dramatic differences in protein and sugar content.

	OIKOS PLAIN GREEK YOGURT	DANNON FRUIT ON THE BOTTOM BLUEBERRY YOGURT
Container size	5.3 oz	6 oz
Calories	80	150
Fat	0 g	1.5 g
Carbohydrate	6 g	29 g
Sugars	6 g	24 g
Protein	15 g	6 g

You might also want to try Icelandic-style *skyr,* a kind of strained yogurt. The brand Siggi's does a good job of minimizing the sugar content, even in flavored yogurt. Whenever possible, choose unflavored yogurt and add some berries.

PROTEIN FROM MEAT

Beef, pork, and game are high-quality, iron-rich sources of protein, but many cuts can also be high in unhealthy fats and calories. Opt for leaner cuts, as well as smaller portions. Good cuts include eye of round, top round, and bottom round, either as a roast or a steak. Use ground sirloin tip or top sirloin for burgers. Most pork (but not bacon) is leaner today than it used to be. Lamb tends to have a high fat content, but there are cuts that pass muster. In general, the tenderloin, loin chops, and leg are the leaner cuts in pork and lamb. Other lean alternatives include game meats such as bison, ostrich, and venison.

THE INCREDIBLE, EDIBLE EGG

The protein in an egg is considered to be perfect, because it has all the essential amino acids and is easy to digest and absorb. In fact, the original gold standard that determined protein quality was based on how well other foods' protein compared to that of an egg. Eggs are incredibly versatile and easy to prepare. My favorite breakfast is an egg-white omelet with one egg yolk, some Hass avocado, and a couple of slices of high-fiber bread. Egg whites contain about half the protein content of the egg. The yolk contains the other half, along with vitamins, minerals, and one essential amino acid, which makes the egg a complete protein. That's why I usually use a single yolk in my omelet. Why do I throw out the rest of the yolks? A large egg contains 80 calories, much of them from the fat in the yolk, and 6 grams of protein. To get enough protein in a meal, I'd need to have five eggs for my omelet, which would add up to about 400 calories. That wouldn't allow me to eat anything else at that meal. If you're uncomfortable tossing egg yolks, look for separated liquid egg whites from Eggology and Egg Beaters in your supermarket.

VEGETABLE PROTEINS

Vegetarians get the majority of their protein from beans, lentils, and other legumes (as well as nuts). Tofu, of course, is made from soybeans. (We'll talk more about legumes on page 17, when we discuss sources of fibrous carbohydrates.) Vegetable proteins also tend to be very high in fiber, which is both a curse and a blessing. Vegetable proteins are good for our digestive health and help with satiety. However, the fiber in legumes makes the protein in these foods slightly less bioavailable. Also, most vegetable proteins don't contain all the amino acids necessary to be considered a complete protein. That means you need to eat more of them for your body to get the same amount of protein that it would from a higher-quality source. And then there is the classic problem with beans. As the old ditty goes, "Beans, beans, the musical fruit. The more you eat, the more you toot!" If eating legumes makes you feel bloated or gassy, an enzyme-based supplement such as Beano can help.

Start Your Day with Protein

The first mistake all too many people watching their weight make is to skip breakfast. The second is to fill up on toast, cereal, donuts, bagels, and other starchy carbohydrates and to ignore protein-packed foods. Sufficient protein at the first meal of the day is crucial to weight management. Why? After you fast all night (that's why it's called break*fast*), consuming protein in the morning provides an initial and sustained feeling of fullness—even more so than when it's consumed at other times during the day.[42] Eating breakfast, particularly one that's high in protein, has been shown to increase the feeling of comfortable fullness and improve the diet quality of overweight teenage girls who had formerly skipped breakfast. It also improved their overall self-control around food and their motivation to avoid overeating.[43]

The *quality* of protein consumed at breakfast is as important as the quantity.[44] In one study, researchers divided overweight subjects into two groups. For a week, both groups ate a breakfast with a similar number of calories and ratio of macronutrients; in other words, the quantity of protein was the same for both groups. But one group consumed a high-quality protein breakfast that included eggs, while the other group ate a lower-quality protein breakfast that included cereal. After 2 weeks, each group was served the other breakfast, again for a week. Those who ate the egg breakfasts felt significantly fuller than they did after eating the cereal breakfasts. Those who ate the egg breakfast also had higher levels of a gut hormone peptide that signals the brain to stop eating, an effect that lasted for a week.

NOT JUST FOR BODYBUILDERS

Protein powder—or protein isolate, as it's also called—is an excellent source of amino acids. Your body quickly absorbs most kinds. So protein powder is an ideal ingredient in smoothies, which are perfect for breakfast. Whey protein also boosts levels of serotonin, the calming, feel-good hormone. Supplementing with whey protein powder can lower both LDL ("bad") and total cholesterol levels and improve insulin levels in heavy people.[45] Many brands and types of protein powder are available, but be sure to use an unsweetened product. My favorites are made from these sources:

- Dairy (whey or casein)
- Soy (non GMO)
- Egg white (albumen)
- Pea

THE IMPORTANCE
OF CARBOHYDRATES

Carbohydrates are an essential component of a healthy diet. Here's why:

- They're the body's preferred source of energy. You can also burn fat for energy, but only after carbohydrate (sugar) has been burned.

- They're a boundless source of vitamins, minerals, and other micronutrients.

- They're contained in a wide array of fruits, vegetables, and grains, helping you add variety and interest to meals and avoid culinary boredom, which can sabotage any weight-loss program.

- They're the only source of fiber (protein and fat have none).

- Those high in fiber help boost satiety, so you actually feel the need to eat less.

GOOD-FOR-YOU CARBS

Carbohydrates have taken a lot of abuse over the past decade. Many significantly low-carb diets have become popular in recent years, and for good reason: Carbohydrates tend to be the one food group we overeat. Moreover,

My Six Go-To Sauces

These condiments add tons of flavor with minimal calorie impact and no fat. To bring interest and pleasing texture to meals, I recommend the following:

1. Balsamic vinegar

2. Mustard, particularly Gulden's Spicy Brown. Avoid products with honey or other sugars.

3. Salsa without added sugar. Check out Pace, Old El Paso, or Newman's Own.

4. Hot sauce, such as Sriracha, Tabasco, or Cholula

5. Lemon juice

6. Worcestershire sauce, such as Lea & Perrins

we generally opt for the wrong carbohydrates. So rather than dwelling on the wrong carbs, let's define what makes a good carbohydrate. It's a five-letter word and it starts with *f*. That's right. Fiber!

Fiber differentiates the carbs we should be eating more of from those we should avoid. First of all, those carbohydrates highest in fiber also tend to be the highest in healthy micronutrients. Take vegetables, fruits, and whole grains. The addition of fiber to a carbohydrate not only makes it more difficult to overeat, but also has a built-in penalty if you do overeat it—namely, gastric distress. This is actually a self-monitoring factor. (The carbs we tend to overeat, though, are essentially void of fiber.)

In this book, I'll refer to the carbs you'll be eating as fibrous carbohydrates, which will make up 50 percent of your calorie intake. Research shows that individuals who take in at least half their calories from carbohydrates are the least likely to be obese.[46] People who've registered on the National Weight Control Registry have maintained an average weight loss of 30 pounds for about 5½ years. On average, they consume about 56 percent of their energy as carbohydrates.[47, 48]

One of the benefits of eating fibrous carbohydrates is that they keep your blood sugar levels low and therefore don't initiate an insulin response. Chronic high insulin levels make us vulnerable to converting and storing

The Staff of Life

I understand how tasty and convenient a couple of slices of toast with your omelet in the morning can be. And in fact, the Scandinavian countries, where bread is a daily staple, are among the healthiest in the world. But there is bread, and then there is bread. I have a simple rule when it comes to choosing whether to eat a particular bread: If a slice contains less than 100 calories and has at least 4 grams of fiber and 3 grams of protein, go for it. Otherwise, steer clear. You can also get your grains from tortillas, crackers, and flatbreads made with sprouted whole grains. (These can usually be found in the health food section of the supermarket.) Nature's Own Double Fiber Wheat bread is a home run with 50 calories per slice, 5 grams of fiber, and 3 grams of protein. Fitness Bread by Mestermacher and Food for Life Ezekiel 4:9 breads, English muffins, and tortillas are also good high-fiber choices.

foods as body fat. In fact, insulin is known as the fat-storage hormone. In recent decades, prediabetes and diabetes have become epidemic, not just in the United States but also throughout the world, paralleling the increase in overweight and obesity. But you needn't become a part of this dangerous trend. Eat carbs full of fiber and follow the whole My 5 Plan, and you'll tame the high blood sugar/excess insulin monster, if not keep it from ever rearing its ugly head.

FIBROUS CARBOHYDRATES ON THE MENU

You'll be focusing on fibrous carbohydrates as you put your meals together, specifically:

- Vegetables

- Fruit

- Whole grains, including high-fiber breads and pastas

- Beans, lentils, and other legumes

You can have all the *non-starchy* fibrous carbohydrates you want at each meal, but you'll limit the amount of starchy ones. (See "What's a Starchy Vegetable?" on page 16.)

Fewer than one in 10 Americans consume the amount of fruits and vegetables recommended by the US Department of Agriculture despite clear evidence of the health benefits of doing so.[49] A new study provides powerful evidence of the importance of eating fruit and vegetables. Researchers reviewed data on the habits and health status of 65,000 British adults collected over an average of 7½ years and found a strong association between produce consumption and reduced risk of death from all causes.[50] Statistically, vegetables slightly beat out fruit.

VEGETABLES are full of micronutrients, and those with the most vibrant, bright colors boast the most of them. They're also great high-volume, low-calorie choices. Take a tip from the Japanese, who try to eat foods of five different colors at each meal, primarily vegetables. It's their way

What's a Starchy Vegetable?

The poor potato often bore the brunt of the prejudice against carbohydrates in the anti-carb craze. But a small baked potato with skin contains only 128 calories and not quite 2 grams of sugar, while delivering 3.5 grams of protein and 3 grams of fiber. It also provides 22 percent of our daily vitamin C requirement, and is a good source of potassium and vitamin B6. There's definitely a place for starchy vegetables in the My 5 Plan, although you'll limit their portion size as you will with whole grains, fruit, lentils, and beans. (Again, you can eat as many non-starchy fibrous veggies as you wish.) Starchy vegetables include:

- Beets
- Carrots (when cooked)
- Corn
- Parsnips
- Plantain
- Pumpkin

- Sweet potato
- Taro
- White potato
- Winter squash
- Yam

of getting a multivitamin. Following their example, you could make a rainbow of a salad with red radishes, yellow peppers, purple cabbage, and orange carrots atop green baby spinach. Keep leafy greens in your fridge for salads. Frozen and canned vegetables are another great choice—and are extremely convenient. Canned tomato paste actually provides more bioavailable lycopene, a micronutrient that may prevent against cancer and heart disease, than do fresh tomatoes.[51]

FRUIT, whether as a snack or part of a meal, is important to My 5. When I researched my book *The 5-Factor World Diet*, I found that the six countries with the highest obesity rates consumed exclusively fruits with a very low fiber content. (See "What Makes a Fruit High Fiber?" opposite.) You'll want to eat primarily high-fiber fruits. Whenever possible, buy fruits that are in season and that are locally grown. However, frozen berries and other fruits are lifesavers, especially off-season, when prices of fresh fruit soar.

WHOLE GRAINS are a great source of soluble fiber and help create a feeling of fullness. Ideally, you want to eat grains that have been minimally processed whenever possible. For example, eating whole quinoa is a better choice than eating bread made from quinoa flour. Typically, when a whole grain is ground, its fibrous shell, and therefore much of its nutritional value, is discarded, although there are some exceptions. Certain breads and pastas on the market today manage to pack a fiber wallop, making them good choices in your diet. Whole grains include whole wheat, brown rice, steel-cut and rolled oats (not the instant kind), barley, wild rice, buckwheat, and Kamut. Quinoa is actually the seed of a leafy plant, rather than a grain, but is treated as a grain. In terms of portion size, treat grains as starchy fibrous carbohydrates.

LENTILS, BEANS, AND OTHER LEGUMES are excellent sources of fiber, as well as protein and healthy fats. Lentils come in red, yellow, green, brown, and black varieties. Other legumes include chickpeas (garbanzos) and black, kidney, navy, pinto, and numerous other beans. Tofu is made

What Makes a Fruit High Fiber?

To achieve your goal of shedding 5 pounds fast, you want to mainly consume fruits that have edible skin or seeds. Not only is that where the fiber is, but it's also where the vitamins and minerals are. Fruits with high-fiber content also contribute to satiety. Here's how to distinguish between the two:

MORE FIBER:	LESS FIBER:
Apple	Mango
Pear	Papaya
Peach or nectarine	Banana
Plum	Grapes
Berries	Pineapple
Cherries	Cantaloupe
Kiwifruit	Honeydew melon
Oranges and other citrus	Watermelon

from fermented soybeans. (Green beans, peas, snow peas, and other fresh vegetables are considered vegetables, rather than legumes, so portions aren't limited.) Canned lentils and other beans are a great convenience. Do rinse them before adding them to salads, soups, or stir-fries to remove the salty liquid in which they've been preserved as well as the color preservative EDTA. In terms of portion size, treat lentils and other legumes as starchy fibrous carbohydrates.

My Favorite Whole Grains

The process that produces refined grains such as white flour removes most of the fiber and many of the micronutrients. Whole grains are a much better way to meet the high-fiber carbohydrate component of your meals. Here are some of my favorites:

1. OATS. Nothing beats a bowl of hot oatmeal on a chilly morning, especially when you serve it with a dollop of Greek yogurt, which is a great source of protein, and some berries. Oats combine soluble and insoluble fiber and are a particularly good source of beta-glucan, a kind of fiber with especially powerful cholesterol-lowering effects that may also boost immune-system function. Check the label. Some oats are processed to cook quickly, which strips them of their fiber.

2. WILD RICE. Nuttier and chewier than white or brown rice, wild rice also contains more protein, fiber, iron, and copper than either.

3. QUINOA. Native to the Andes, quinoa is technically a pseudo-grain. Gluten-free, it's the only vegetarian source of complete protein. One-third cup of cooked quinoa contains 3 grams of fiber. Quinoa cooks in half the time rice does.

4. RYE. This grain has a hearty taste and valuable micronutrient content. Most rye bread is made of wheat flour with a bit of rye flour thrown in; 100 percent rye pumpernickel is a better choice. Crisp crackers made of 100 percent rye or mixed with other grains are widely available.

5. WHEAT BERRIES. Flour is milled from wheat berries, but the berry itself retains all of its nutrients and has a wonderfully nutty flavor. Cook and serve as a breakfast cereal or side dish, or toss with cut-up vegetables and dress with olive oil and vinegar for a satisfying salad.

GALA

LEA

xxxxxxx8342

. 11/1/2021

Item: ï¿½0010086060851 ((book)

A Glimpse at the Glycemic Index

A few years ago, the glycemic index (GI) was popping up all over the place as the key to weight loss. (You'll recall that I studied under the two professors who pioneered this research.) *Glycemic* refers to sugar, and the GI is the relative speed with which eating a certain portion of any carbohydrate food raises your blood sugar level, as measured on a scale of 1 to 100. High-GI foods are apt to stimulate insulin, the fat-storing hormone, and to stall your weight-loss efforts. I don't talk much about the GI in this book, because it doesn't take into consideration portion size or other foods being consumed at the same time—what's known as the glycemic load of a meal. So while the GI may be meaningful in a lab, it isn't when it comes to a meal made up of protein and fat, along with carbohydrates. For example, white rice has a really high GI, but if you're serving it with a stir-fry of shrimp and veggies topped with a slice of avocado, its glycemic impact is actually very low. That's what we're talking about in this book—the *gestalt*, the big picture. All too often we zero in on single activities and single foods and we miss the big picture.

FIBER AND WEIGHT LOSS

Fiber is a crucial component of the My 5 Plan. Most Americans don't consume enough of either of the two types of fiber, soluble and insoluble, both of which are essential for good health.[52] (See "Soluble and Insoluble Fiber" on page 20.) In addition to aiding digestion and regularity, fiber plays an important role in preventing many diseases, including heart disease,[53] colon cancer,[54] and stroke.[55]

Fiber is also an effective tool for weight management because it fills us up quickly despite having very few calories. Low intake of fiber and high intake of fat are associated with excess weight.[56] The American Heart Association recommends a daily consumption of 25 to 30 grams of fiber to help stem the high incidence of overweight and obesity.[57] Here's how fiber helps you lose fat pounds:

Soluble and Insoluble Fiber

	FOUND PRIMARILY IN	ACTION	BENEFITS
Insoluble Fiber	Whole grains, vegetables	Cannot be digested	Scrubs intestinal wall; aids satiety
Soluble Fiber	Seeds, nuts, oat bran, fruit	Dissolves in water; digestible	Prolongs digestion time, prolonging fullness; lowers LDL ("bad") cholesterol

- It slows digestion, helping to even out blood sugar levels. High blood sugar can spike an insulin response, which can encourage your body to store fat.

- It keeps blood sugar on a steady plane, helping control appetite.

- It maintains healthy insulin levels, minimizing the likelihood of developing diabetes or heart disease, which are associated with obesity.

- It provides satiety, a comfortable feeling of fullness, helping mute hunger, curb cravings for sweet and starchy foods, and generally reduce food intake, resulting in weight loss.

Follow the meal plans for My 5 found on page 126 and you'll be consuming the amount of fiber recommended by the American Heart Association.

Super Seeds

They may be small, but seeds are packed with healthy fats, protein, and fiber, all of which contribute to satiety, making them helpful for weight loss. (They also boast a host of vitamins and minerals.) But there's a big caveat about seeds: Like nuts, they're sky-high in calories, so petite portions are in order. Two tablespoons of pumpkin seeds (pepitas) make a portable snack. Seeds also add flavor and texture to your meals. Add a tablespoon of sesame or chia seeds to a bowl of oatmeal or sprinkle a few pumpkin or sunflower seeds on a salad or stir-fry. Add a tablespoon of chia seeds or ground flaxseed to a smoothie.

THE HEALTHY FATS

In the 1980s and '90s, the media did its best to scare us off of eating fats of any kind. The message was that eliminating dietary fat, which has more than twice as many calories per gram as protein or carbohydrates, would banish body fat. Millions of fat-free Snackwell's cookies and Red Vines licorice sticks later, we've come to realize that replacing fat with sugar is not the answer. Further, a large body of scientific research has taught us how essential dietary fat is to both our health and our waistlines. Scientists discovered that eating certain dietary fats, including salmon and other fatty

The Skinny on Fats

	TYPE OF FAT	SOURCES	SPECIFIC FOODS	COMMENTS
Eat	Monounsaturated	Vegetables and nuts	Olive and canola oils; walnuts and other nuts; avocado; olives	Liquid at room temperature
Eat	Polyunsaturated	Vegetables, seeds, some nuts, and fatty fish	Corn, sunflower, high-oleic safflower, flaxseed, and grape-seed oils; fatty fish such as sardines, salmon, and herring	Liquid at room temperature
Limit	Saturated	Primarily meat and dairy products	Beef, poultry, pork, bacon, butter, coconut oil, lard, palm oil	Solid at room temperature
Avoid	Trans fats	Processed foods; deep-fried foods	Almost all commercially baked and other processed foods once contained trans fats, but many have now eliminated them.	Check ingredient lists. May appear as "hydrogenated oil" or "partially hydrogenated oil"

Five Reasons to Eat Healthy Fats

1. They promote satiety, which helps suppress your appetite. Add fat to your meal and you'll feel fuller longer.[58, 59]

2. They help your body absorb the fat-soluble vitamins A, D, E, and K.[60]

3. They help burn body fat and reduce fat deposition.[61]

4. They provide a major source of energy to the body. One-third cup of nuts or 2 tablespoons of peanut butter contains the same energy as a 1-ounce serving of cooked lean meat.[62]

5. Omega-3 fatty acids foster production of certain hormones.[63]

fish, olives and olive oil, avocados, and nuts and seeds, actually helps us burn body fat.

Just as with carbohydrates, there are certain fats we want to minimize in our diet and other fats we can maximize. Monounsaturated and polyunsaturated fats are part of a healthy diet. The essential fatty acids omega-3 and omega-6 are a subset of polyunsaturated fats; *essential* means that your body cannot manufacture them so we must get them from our food. Minimize saturated fats, found in meat and most other animal foods, which contribute to heart disease. Trans

My Five Favorite Fats

1. Hass avocado. *Interesting fact:* If you put avocado on your burger or ham sandwich, it lowers the inflammation markers from the meat.[64]

2. Almonds. *Interesting fact:* When eaten in moderation, almonds can help achieve weight loss.[65]

3. Olive oil. *Interesting fact:* Extra-virgin olive oil is more likely to induce satiety after a meal than other oils.[66]

4. Wild salmon. *Interesting fact:* Two 3-ounce servings of salmon a week can raise HDL ("good") cholesterol levels.[67]

5. Pumpkin seeds. *Interesting fact:* Native Americans traditionally used pumpkin seeds to treat kidney problems and eliminate intestinal parasites.

fats, found in deep-fried foods and many packaged pastries, are associated with various cancers. The labeling regulations on trans fats are a bit confusing, but as long as you don't eat these foods, there's no need to look at their labels. (For more on the different kinds of fats, review "The Skinny on Fats" on page 21.)

DRINK UP

Staying hydrated is always important, but all the more so when you're burning your body fat for energy. Most people are borderline dehydrated at all times. It's easy to confuse hunger with thirst, so sip frequently and your apparent hunger may vanish. The best beverage of all is water. I suggest women drink about 8 cups a day and men about 10 cups. Just add a spritz of lemon or lime juice if you wish. Some of your intake can come from other beverages, including chicken broth and other clear soups and the following drinks:

- Tea, whether caffeinated, decaffeinated, or herbal
- Coffee, both decaffeinated and caffeinated (limit to 3 cups a day)
- Sparkling water
- Naturally sweetened calorie-free flavored beverages such as vitaminwater zero or fruitwater.

If you follow my rule that you eat calories, but you don't *drink* calories, you'll understand why fruit juice isn't on the list. Containing neither protein, fat, nor fiber, fruit juice is calorically dense, provides no satiety, and receives 100 percent of its calories from sugar. Just compare a cup of unsweetened apple juice with a medium-size apple: The former contains 114 calories and zero fiber; the latter has only about 72 calories but boasts 3.5 grams of fiber.

MOVING FORWARD

Now that you've read this chapter, you have a good idea of what you'll be eating over the next 5 days. But I want to make this really simple for you. In Chapter 6, "The 5-Day Diet," we'll move from the conceptual to the actual.

There you'll find a day-by-day diet guide, complete with meal plans, portion guidelines, snack ideas, and foods to have on hand at all times, all designed to make eating the My 5 way easy, enjoyable, filling—and delicious.

Although the premise (and the promise) of this book is that you'll lose 5 pounds in 5 days—and you will if you follow all five guidelines and don't stray when it comes to your meals and snacks—this is far more than a quickie weight-loss book or a quickie diet. It's also about leading an active lifestyle, getting enough sleep, and detaching yourself for at least a while from the TV, computer, and other electronics that increasingly rule our lives. Nor is it just about just 5 days. To allow your body to keep changing over time, the program will keep evolving, increasing the array of ingredients in recipes, changing up the workout exercises, and responding to other variables, all of which we'll discuss in Part II.

Meanwhile, read on to explore the second component of my revolutionary program: Five minutes of resistance exercise each day.

Five Key Points in Chapter 1

1. Eat three meals a day (composed of protein, fibrous carbohydrates, and healthy fats), along with two snacks (composed of protein and fibrous carbohydrates), using your hand to judge portion sizes and following the meal plans on page 126.

2. Never allowing yourself to get super hungry will help you control your appetite and eliminate cravings so you lose weight more quickly.

3. Eating protein at every meal and for each snack preserves lean muscle even as you lose fat, and also aids satiety. A protein-rich breakfast helps reduce overall calorie intake over the whole day.

4. All carbohydrates are not created equal. Eat primarily fiber-rich carbohydrates, such as vegetables, fruits, whole grains, and lentils and other beans, which help fill you up. Fibrous carbohydrates also help moderate your blood sugar and insulin levels, so you're less likely to store body fat.

5. Healthy fats are essential for your body to function properly. They also play a key role in weight loss because they make you feel full longer. Plus, they help burn body fat and reduce fat storage.

FLEX YOUR MUSCLES DAILY

The word *exercise* has become far too broad and generic. No wonder. You might walk around the block and proudly report, "I just got some exercise." Your brother might do some powerlifting and call that exercise, while your husband might run wind sprints and call them exercise. Your mom might call her yoga session exercise. Yes, each of these activities and many others are forms of contrived exercise. In turn, they fall into two primary categories: resistance exercise and aerobic activity. But another, often underappreciated kind of activity, referred to as "chronic movement," comprises the activities that make up daily life, such as going to the mailbox, climbing stairs, and making dinner. Another mouthful of a name for chronic movement is non-exercise activity thermogenesis, or NEAT, which we'll discuss in the next chapter.

I like to say that we exercise too much and move too little. How come? Because we attach such importance to exercise ("Gotta get to the gym") and so little importance to moving ("I'll walk to meet my friends at the restaurant"). Admit it, we all spend too many hours sacked out on the couch.

Engaging in *both* exercise and movement will help you lose those first (or last) 5 pounds on the My 5 Plan. In addition to helping manage your weight, the combination of both resistance and aerobic exercise offers many other health benefits. In this chapter we'll talk about resistance exercise; in the next chapter, we'll cover movement in general and walking in particular.

WHAT EXACTLY IS RESISTANCE EXERCISE?

Resistance exercise goes by several other names: resistance training, strength training, weight-bearing exercise, and weight training. I prefer the first term, which is more descriptive and precise. In this type of exercise, a muscle or muscle group works against a certain resistance for a short period of time. Performance is limited to the fatigue of that muscle or those muscle groups, known as local fatigue. Using dumbbells or doing Pilates, certain forms of yoga, and body-weight resistance exercises (such as planks and lunges) are all examples of resistance exercise. In the case of lunges, pushups, Pilates, and some forms of yoga, your own body weight provides the resistance.

Using weights, a.k.a. weight training, is one kind of resistance exercise. Instead of your own body weight providing resistance, dumbbells do the job—with your help, of course. While both body-weight resistance and dumbbells (or other free weights) have their unique benefits, including balance, stress relief, and flexibility, the truth is that the use of free weights remains the most intense and delivers the most dramatic and immediate results. The exercises you'll be doing as part of My 5 include both weight training and body resistance.

FORGET THESE MISCONCEPTIONS

Do the terms *workout, hit the gym,* and *pump some iron* make you cringe? Do you immediately envision muscle-bound bodybuilders lifting giant weights, CrossFit fanatics flipping humungous tires, or the world's strong-man competitors pulling cars across a field? Like many people, you may have a lot of preconceived ideas about resistance exercise, like these:

- It takes hours of working out to see results.
- It involves intense circuits of power-lifting heavy weights.
- It requires working out in a gym on fancy machines.
- It can make women overly muscular and bulky.
- It requires lots of pain for little gain.

This may explain why, according to the Centers for Disease Control and Prevention, only 19 percent of women do resistance training two or more times a week. Forget all that.

Instead, I'm proposing a revolutionary approach to resistance exercise. Here's why it's revolutionary:

- You can do it anywhere, even in the privacy of your home.
- All you need are a few inexpensive dumbbells.
- It takes only about 5 minutes a day to see results in the form of a toned, sleeker body! Yes, you read that right: 5 minutes!
- Women needn't worry about developing bulging muscles. No way on 5 minutes a day.
- And most of all, forget the whole idea of "no pain, no gain." That's just another way of describing an injury waiting to happen.

MINIMUM TIME, MAXIMUM RESULTS

Now let's zero in on the old excuse you've probably used in the past: I just don't have time to fit this into my busy life. Once you understand that you can get all the benefits of resistance exercise in *as little as 5 minutes* a day, that old excuse won't fly! During my early years as a trainer, I struggled with this challenge of how to attain lasting results without a huge investment of time. I've always known how to get results for my clients, but I also realized that the time commitment involved was a turnoff for many people.

Then, as I was researching my last book, *The Body Reset Diet,* I had a moment of clarity that made me rethink our current weight-loss paradigm: move more and eat less. I realized that people were able to lose weight on many different diets, yet almost all of them regained that weight and sometimes more. So, as I mentioned earlier, with the help of a few very talented scientists, I spent the past couple of years collecting and analyzing data on weight-loss habits, techniques, and behaviors.

I discovered that there are other integral components of the weight-loss process in addition to dieting. If you integrate them into your weight-loss program, the dieting process itself needn't be so drastic or extreme. Basically, it comes down to what's the *least* amount you need to diet if you're doing all the other things right? And then what *are* those other things?

During this research phase I also interviewed professional bodybuilders. I remembered reading an article by Arnold Schwarzenegger about the early days of physique sculpting when he lived in Austria. Every few months he and his fellow bodybuilders would put a bar and some weight plates into the back of a van and drive to the countryside. There they'd take turns doing one exercise, such as a squat or deadlift, until they could no longer stand. Don't worry—I'm not recommending this. But I was fascinated by the idea that a workout could be only one exercise. After their exertions, Arnold and his buddies would have dinner around a campfire, fall asleep, and head home in the morning. The truth is, you can profoundly change your body with one exercise a day.

I looked at the many reasons that people choose not to do resistance exercise or choose not to continue with it and found these five stumbling blocks:

1. They don't have the time.

2. They don't have or can't afford a gym membership.

3. They don't have the know-how to do a complex program.

4. They're intimidated by the images they see in infomercials for workouts such as Insanity P90X.

5. They have been injured or are afraid of getting injured.

TIME IS OF THE ESSENCE

As I assembled the pieces of the puzzle, two key points emerged strong and loud. First, short, intense workouts are more effective than longer workouts, which focus on endurance.[1, 2] Second, variation is as essential as intensity for the most efficient workout.[3-5] Plus, it keeps things interesting, enhancing adherence. I combined these two fitness "truths" into an easy-to-follow, time-sensitive approach that delivers immediate results. The answer: short, frequent workouts.

Unlike traditional resistance exercise, where you go the gym, perform many different exercises, and call it a workout, my revolutionary approach bucks that old paradigm. Instead, I've simplified and optimized the essence of resistance exercise by answering these two questions:

1. What are the *most effective* exercises necessary to achieve the greatest results?

2. What is the *least amount* of exercise you need to do to maximize results?

I needn't remind you that time is perhaps our most precious commodity these days. The idea is to lower the bar regarding resistance exercise—a bar that's unnecessarily high at the moment—without sacrificing a great outcome. The program introduced in this book does just that. It allows you to focus on just one exercise a day. That's it! No need to pack your gym bag and drive to the gym. No need to change into workout gear. And if you have young kids, no need to get a sitter or bundle them up and take them to the gym's childcare room.

This is a way of doing resistance exercise that you've likely never done before. The key to the whole My 5 Plan is to simplify and optimize, both in your meals and in your approach to exercise. To change your muscles and your metabolism (which, of course, helps you lose weight), you need to create enough intensity, enough focus, and enough volume to stress those muscles. And that's why we do one exercise a day focusing on one body part. With intensity and focus, you get the job done—fast.

Don't worry about overdoing resistance training if exercising every day. Remember, it's only 5 minutes or so. Just as you'll be eating well *every day*, without taking the weekend off, your activity level should be consistent from day to day as it evolves into a daily habit. Doing a little bit every single day is way more impactful than doing a lot some days and nothing other days. And it's important to remember that you'll never be working the same muscle group on consecutive days. This is a 5-day program, and while it's not possible to work all the muscle groups, one at a time, in just 5 days, you *can* do so in a week. That means you'll complete the cycle on the following 2 days, and repeat the sequence starting on Day 8.

Do you brush your hair only 4 days a week? Do you brush your teeth only 5 days a week? Do you eat dinner only 3 nights a week? Of course not. Certain behaviors are permanent, perpetual, and daily. Likewise, all five behaviors integral to My 5 will become part of your daily life, including the resistance exercises. On conventional programs, you generally work out only 2 or 3 days a week because the exercises are long, are exhausting, involve equipment, and typically require you go somewhere like a gym or studio. But in this revolutionary program, the bar is so low—only a single exercise for approximately 5 minutes a day—it will easily become part of your daily routine.

IS 5 MINUTES TOO GOOD TO BE TRUE?

Much as you may love the idea that I'm asking you to commit to only 5 minutes of resistance exercise a day, there may be a little nagging voice in the back of your mind saying, "How can that little bit of time possibly help me lose fat pounds and gain more muscle?" Here's my promise. Give it 5 days, and you'll begin to see a difference in your energy level and your weight.

The resistance exercise component of My 5 optimizes efficiency, in terms of time and results, by combining the two fitness principles of variety and intensity. Here's another reason it's so effective: Many other fitness programs are so grueling that it's easy to make excuses to skip a day when you're tired or sick. Do that too often, and before you know it, you've lost your momentum, along with your commitment to stick with the program. My 5-minute approach is the only kind of workout that you can still do even when you feel a cold coming on or otherwise aren't quite up to snuff. That's a major plus, because research shows that short, moderately intense workouts can improve immune system function, while longer workouts may overtax the immune system.[6–9]

MINIMUM OUTPUT, MAXIMUM RETURN

My approach to resistance exercise is just revolutionary—and it works. I know that because I've prescribed it to hundreds of my clients and they've experienced the kind of fabulous (and fast) results you want. After all, the reason many people don't stay with a resistance exercise program is the perceived time commitment. But don't just rely on my word. Loads of research supports the fact that doing the right exercises on a regular basis for short but intense periods can be highly effective. (It's also a lot safer than longer exercise sessions.) Let's look at a few of the studies.

To determine if 1 set of resistance exercises can be as effective as 3 sets, researchers studied men in their late teens and early twenties. The subjects, who had been resistance training recreationally for a year or more, were divided into two groups. One group did one set of 6 repetitions, and the other group did 3 sets of upper-body resistance exercises until they could do no more. Both groups followed their regimen three times a week. Researchers measured the subjects' muscular strength and body fat before the study and at its conclusion, 8 weeks later, and found that both groups had increased their strength about equally.[10] But interestingly, despite spending almost 70 percent less time exercising, the 1-set group showed a significantly greater reduction in body fat than the 3-set group. Other studies support this conclusion. The takeaway? Both beginner and recreational strength trainers can benefit from short but intense periods of exercise.

Such benefits can continue to accrue over time. In another study, researchers also compared the value of different amounts of resistance exercise, but this time the subjects had been recreational weight lifters for about 6 years and had been performing 1 set of a nine-exercise resistance-training circuit for at least 1 year. Both groups did the circuit-training program three times a week, but one group performed 1 set and the other group 3 sets, both of 8 to 12 reps, until their muscles were fatigued. The first group took about 25 minutes, and the second about 1 hour. After 13 weeks, both groups had significantly improved their muscular strength, endurance, and body composition (amount of body fat). This means that one-set programs are still effective even after a year of training. And it also shows that increasing training volume doesn't lead to significantly greater improvements in fitness.[11]

Another study reveals that doing one set of resistance exercises that requires only 15 minutes to complete was as effective as doing three sets of resistance exercises that required 35 minutes to complete.[12] Despite taking more than twice as long, the latter approach didn't show an advantage in raising the subjects' resting metabolic rate, which was significantly higher in both groups, even 72 hours later. Subjects in both groups continued to burn roughly an additional 100 calories a day. This means that following the American College of Sports Medicine guidelines for resistance training to provide overall muscular fitness is also enough to offset increases in fat mass, and therefore weight gain, for the vast majority of people.

In another study, researchers used the same subjects to explore the different effects on weight control by increasing their resting metabolic rate. The men were divided into two groups. On one day, one group followed a high-intensity interval resistance training (HIRT) protocol, while the other group completed the traditional resistance training protocol. On another day, each group performed the alternative exercise.[13] For the HIRT part of the test, the men did a total of 7 sets of three exercises with 20- to 30-second rests between sets. For the traditional part of the test, they did eight exercises for a total of 32 sets with 1- or 2-minute rests between sets. Twenty-two hours after they completed each protocol, the men's resting metabolic rate and respiratory ratio were measured. The shorter sessions increased the men's resting energy expenditure to a greater extent than traditional resistance training did. It also reduced their respiratory rate, allowing them to burn a larger amount of fat at rest.

While these studies used subjects already accustomed to resistance training, overweight adults have also shown positive results from shorter resistance training sessions. In one study, overweight, formerly sedentary young adults engaged in three weekly resistance exercise sessions of 11 minutes each, while a similar control group did not exercise. After 6 months, the exercisers had significantly increased the number of calories burned each day and increased their lean muscle mass by almost 3 percent. The exercisers also saw their resting metabolism increase significantly. The authors concluded that even short sessions of regular resistance training can help prevent obesity in at-risk young adults.[14]

Other studies have concluded that as little as 20 minutes of whole-body resistance training two or three times a week, in keeping with American College of Sports Medicine guidelines,[15] could reduce abdominal fat and increase resting metabolism.[16] [17] Moreover, 2 months of resistance exercise was shown to have the potential to reverse about 20 years' worth of the loss of strength and muscle mass normally associated with aging.[18]

It also turns out that several brief, "snack-size" portions of exercise are more effective at controlling blood sugar than a single, continuous workout. (Remember, keeping blood sugar on an even keel helps moderate your appetite and enables your body to burn fat.) A recent New Zealand study first had insulin-resistant volunteers (meaning their blood sugar tended to peak after meals) walk on a treadmill for half an hour before dinner. After several days, the subjects worked out on the treadmill before breakfast, lunch, and dinner in snack-size portions. Each time, they strolled for 1 minute, followed by 1 minute of fast walking, and so on, for 12 minutes. At the end of the day, they had completed a *total* of 18 minutes of intense exercise (6 minutes of fast walking three times) each day. Finally, the subjects interspersed resistance band exercises with walking on the treadmill, again in snack-size portions, for 18 minutes of intense exercise. The results? After the 30-minute walk, blood sugar levels were no

The Other Kind of Exercise

Aerobic exercise, also known as cardiovascular exercise, or cardio for short, is basically any activity that involves what fitness experts refer to as moderate-intensity, chronic movement, also known as submaximal chronic movement. So, going for a walk, jogging, cycling, or doing any other activity that raises your heart rate and elevates your metabolism falls into the category of aerobic exercise. The primary distinction between it and resistance exercise is that aerobic exercise is limited by what's called general fatigue. In other words, *you* get tired, rather than fatiguing a specific muscle or muscle group. We'll delve into aerobic activity, primarily in the form of walking, in the next chapter. The two forms of exercise complement each other, and both are important for health and fitness.

lower than they were at the baseline. However, the two snack-size workouts lowered postmeal blood sugar levels, and the effects remained for 24 hours.[19]

BUILDING STRONG MUSCLES

With resistance exercise, you deliberately stress your body's muscle fibers to stimulate them; then, over the next 24 to 72 hours, they recover. And when they heal, they become stronger and denser than they were before. That's why you shouldn't work the same muscles or groups of muscles day after day, but instead allow them to repair and strengthen themselves before they're stimulated again. In this program, each body part has several days to recover as you concentrate on other muscle groups, one day at a time.

Think of resistance exercise much as you do about antibiotics. Both need to be administered for a specific duration, frequency, and intensity. Just as if you were to overconsume antibiotics, overdoing resistance exercise won't necessarily give you a better result. In fact, much like taking extra antibiotics might habituate you to that medication and make it less effective if and when you face a serious infection—or even make you sick by destroying the good bacteria in your digestive tract—overdoing resistance exercise may give you worse results. You may even injure yourself. Again, forget "no pain, no gain!"

That doesn't mean you won't be working hard for 5 minutes. Doing resistance exercise in a sporadic way won't get you results—just as taking that antibiotic for only a few days rather than taking the full course is unlikely to be effective. As with all five of my "prescriptions," your 5-minute resistance training fitness program is an ongoing component of My 5 that will enable you to achieve and then maintain a slim, trim body.

EIGHT REASONS TO DO RESISTANCE EXERCISE

You've probably have heard the old expression that you can kill two birds with one stone, referring to the efficiency of performing two tasks at the same time. Today, we call it multitasking and pride ourselves on making the most of our time. But how about killing *eight* birds with one stone? The benefits of resistance exercise include:

1. Raising your resting metabolism, so you burn more calories at rest and offset your body's tendency to burn fewer calories as you slim down.[20, 21]

2. Protecting existing lean muscle mass and counteracting its atrophy from weight loss or the aging process.[22, 23]

3. Prompting your body to release hormones, including growth hormone and testosterone, which help build new muscle, shaping and sculpting your body so you look leaner, all the while burning fat stores.[24]

4. Increasing bone density. In fact, numerous studies show that following a regular strength-training program can prevent or forestall osteoporosis and may help prevent fractures.[25, 26]

5. Improving balance by using free weights, helping guard against injury, and improving coordination and dexterity.[27]

Five Reasons Why My 5 Resistance Exercises Are Easy to Do

1. You'll do only one each day for only 5 minutes.

2. They're all extremely simple to understand.

3. They don't demand any specific skill set.

4. They require little or no equipment.

5. They can be modified based on your fitness status.

6. Toning your body in a way that helps you look leaner and slimmer.[28, 29]

7. Increasing insulin sensitivity, meaning your body can utilize glucose from carbohydrate consumption more effectively.[30]

8. Increasing your metabolism directly after a workout, known as after-burn, during which you briefly burn additional calories.[31]

Finally, these effects enhance your sense of accomplishment and well-being, which can be a powerful motivator to stay in control of your weight and to continue your resistance exercising. [32, 33] Let's look at some of these effects more closely.

THE BURNING QUESTION OF BURNING CALORIES AT REST

You now know that resistance exercise is about stimulating a specific muscle or muscle group and that it also burns calories. But what you may not have realized is that you don't burn more calories only while you're doing curls or lunges or shoulder presses. In a pair of studies published in 1994, the authors concluded that for every pound of lean muscle tissue, the body burns 50 extra calories a day.[34, 35] But some, including obesity researcher (and my fellow Canadian) Claude Bouchard, PhD, of the Pennington Biomedical Research Center, claim it's far fewer.[36] Regardless, increasing your resting metabolism has been described as the most important result of resistance exercise. As the muscles involved in resistance exercises become stronger and denser, another bonus is that they also cause your body to burn more calories between workouts and even when you're at rest—and that includes sleeping or watching your favorite sitcom.

Without question, the more lean muscle tissue you have, the more effective your metabolism. First of all, your body will be more insulin sensitive, meaning you're less likely to store body fat. You'll have a higher level of growth hormone, which helps build muscle. Your muscles will require more oxygen, burning more calories per movement and per day. Then, depending on which research you believe, you'll burn anywhere from 10 to 50 extra calories per pound of muscle per day. Even at the lowest end, as little as 5 pounds of muscle can help you lose 5 pounds of body fat per year; at the highest end, it could be as much as 50 pounds.

A higher resting metabolism achieved through resistance exercise also explains why men can usually eat more than women of a comparable size and age. Men inherently have more lean muscle tissue, thanks to having more testosterone (and less estrogen) in their bodies than women of comparable age and weight.

RESISTANCE EXERCISE AND INSULIN RESISTANCE

The job of the hormone insulin is to ferry glucose (from carbohydrates) out of your bloodstream and into your fat and muscle cells, where it can be used for energy. However, if your body becomes insulin resistant, entry into the cells is impaired. In addition to the possibility of inducing dangerously high blood sugar levels, insulin resistance means that body fat is stored, instead of metabolized, resulting in weight gain.

What are the ways to address insulin resistance? Losing weight, eating fewer empty carbohydrates, and doing resistance exercises. Combining all three behaviors is ideal. Sounds like My 5! Even a single session of resistance exercise has been shown to increase glucose uptake by cells.[37] Over time, resistance exercise reduces the ratio of fat to lean muscle tissue. And once you've lost weight, resistance exercise helps you maintain your new weight, which in turn benefits insulin sensitivity.[38] You burn fat instead of storing it, which helps you slim down, which in turn benefits insulin sensitivity. This happy outcome is the opposite of a vicious cycle!

PROTECT YOUR LEAN TISSUE

The second most important value of resistance exercise is that it offsets the tendency to lose lean muscle tissue when you reduce your overall intake of calories, as long as you consume enough protein, as you do on My 5. Regular resistance exercise can also counteract any risk of muscle atrophy, which is part of the normal aging process. With a regular program of weight-bearing exercise, you can continue to build muscle well into your ninth decade![39] Speaking of aging, resistance exercise also strengthens bones, so an older person who regularly does weight-bearing exercise is less likely to lose inches in height or suffer fractures, and can actually build bone mass.[40-44]

OFFSET LOWER ENERGY EXPENDITURE

As you slim down, your body burns fewer calories each day. Think about it. A 175-pound guy requires more energy than a 130-pound woman just to power his body's natural processes. Likewise, as you subtract pounds, you naturally expend fewer calories, not just engaging in activities but also powering your human "machine." Regular resistance exercise both increases your resting metabolism and counteracts that reduction in calorie expenditure (as discussed on pages 36–37).

CALORIES IN, CALORIES OUT

Although resistance exercise isn't nearly as effective by itself as it is in combination with a weight-loss diet such as the one introduced in Chapter 1, that combo plus the other three components of My 5 will absolutely erase those first (or last) 5 pounds. [45, 46] More good news: Resistance exercise has conclusively been shown to help you avoid weight regain.[47, 48] And after all, isn't that the last thing you want to happen after you do banish those pesky 5 pounds?

LOOK SLIMMER

Wait, there's more. As if these great results aren't compelling enough, resistance exercise also shapes, tones, and sculpts your body. And that helps you *appear* slimmer. You can actually create the illusion of a longer, leaner body just by strengthening certain muscles with a specific ratio to other muscles. For example, some people overtrain the muscles on the front of their body—what are referred to as mirror muscles. They're the ones you see when

Breathe Correctly

One of the mistakes people new to resistance exercise make is to hold their breath as they perform the exercises. Proper breathing is essential to create power and to not elevate your blood pressure as you exert yourself. So when do you inhale and when do you exhale? Every exercise has two phases: a positive (concentric) phase and a negative (eccentric) one. We do the work during the positive phase, meaning our muscles have to work against gravity. And during the negative phase, gravity does most of the work. If you're ever not sure which is which, just imagine yourself doing the exercise and falling asleep. Where's the weight going to fall? You got it: During the negative phase.

Your objective is to breathe out on the positive phase and in on the negative. An easy way to remember what to do when is to remind yourself to "whistle while you work." Think of the sound karate experts make each time they kick and punch; that's the noise they make as they breathe out when they're doing the work. Ditto for the grunts a sumo wrestler makes. You're doing the same thing, although probably nowhere near as forcefully.

you look directly in the mirror: chest, biceps, front of the abs, and quads. Focusing primarily on those muscle groups closes in your posture by rolling the shoulders forward and bending over from the midsection. You look shorter and stouter and may even appear to have a belly when you don't actually have one. Over-strengthening your front rolls everything forward, bringing you into a hunched-forward position. This is the last thing you want!

Instead, you want to look great from all angles, right? But of course, most of the time you see yourself only from the front. By focusing too much on certain body parts and giving other parts short shrift, you may be compromising your posture, limiting your flexibility, and putting yourself at risk for injury. Instead, you want to work opposing muscle groups equally. For example, your hamstrings oppose your quadriceps; your upper back opposes your chest, and your biceps oppose your triceps. Most people already have stronger anterior (front) muscles than posterior (back) muscles, which is why I like to focus on the back half of the body to correct this imbalance.

If you've ever seen Leonardo da Vinci's "Vitruvian Man" drawing of a man perfectly inscribed within a circle and square, you'll have a great image of what I regard as the ideal posture for men and women. To achieve perfect posture, you need to focus on the posterior muscles of your body. So instead of doing crunches to work on your abs, I'm going to ask you to do the Superman, where you lie on your stomach and raise your arms and legs simultaneously (see page 218).

THE SKINNY ON WEIGHTS

The only equipment you'll initially need to perform the My 5 resistance exercises is a pair of hand weights, also known as free weights or dumbbells. If you're on a tight budget, perhaps you can find dumbbells on Craigslist or at a garage sale. I have no doubt that many weights are sitting unloved and unused in many a garage and basement all across North America! Although you don't need a full set of four different weights when you're getting started, having a lighter pair and a slightly heavier pair is a good idea. You've undoubtedly seen magazine and online articles that suggest using soup cans or detergent bottles filled with water or sand in lieu of dumbbells. Sure, you can do that, but for the sake of this book (and your life), I suggest you take things up a notch by investing in a couple of pairs of the real McCoy.

With dumbbells, you know exactly how many pounds you're lifting, and you can increase this number over time, as we'll discuss in Part II. You'll probably find that you can heft more or less weight depending on the body part you're working. Most people can handle more weight for bicep curls, for example, than for triceps extensions. Or you may be able to do your first set or two of exercises with a heavier weight and then lighten up for the second or third set. That's why it makes sense to have both a lighter and a heavier pair. This also encourages you to use the heavier dumbbells once you've mastered the exercises and built your strength.

The reason I recommend using dumbbells as opposed to exclusively using your body weight for resistance exercise is threefold:

1. Not all body parts can be as effectively worked using your own weight.

2. You can change the weight as you become progressively stronger to make the resistance greater, while you can't change your body weight—at least not in a matter of minutes!

3. Dumbbells are easy to handle and allow natural movement, as each hand can move independently of the other and on multiple planes.

MAKE IT A HABIT

On My 5, your initial resistance exercise "snacks" will be about 5 minutes long, but over time, as you get stronger and build your endurance, you'll want to increase your time commitment, while keeping it to a manageable number of minutes, to maximize results. The great results you'll experience within just a few days will be a powerful motivator to continue this approach to resistance exercise, in concert with the other four new behaviors. And that, of course, is the path to controlling your weight for good. When your behavior rewards you with good results and good feelings, you're well on your way to making it a habit. After all, a habit is just behavior repeated day in and day out. With time, it becomes automatic. Just as you don't think about whether or not to brush your teeth or wash your face, feed your cat or dog, or lock the front door at bedtime, your resistance training program will become one of your regular daily activities.

VARIETY IS THE SPICE OF LIFE

Remember how you felt after you had your first cup of coffee? A year later you moved up to a grande, then a venti. (For those of you who don't frequent Starbucks, that's a medium and a large.) Next thing you knew, you were having two coffees a day just to get the same buzz you got from that first shot of java. Your body gets habituated to a stimulus, whether it's a drug or an exercise. For that reason, it's very important to avoid plateauing, which is why we keep changing the format of that resistance exercise. If you've read my first book, *5-Factor Fitness,* you're familiar with how to manipulate the variables of resistance exercise: the specific exercise you do, the number of repetitions, the number of sets, the level of resistance, and the amount of rest between sets. Your body responds more quickly and consistently when you vary the activity.

I'll show and tell you how to perform seven key exercises that target the main muscle groups we need to address. You can continue to follow this program every single day of your life. It's as simple and efficient as that. Turn to page 216 for photos of yours truly demonstrating the exercises, along with step-by-step instructions. And by the way, if for some reason you cannot do your exercises one day, be sure to catch up the following day by doing two exercises.

Compare my 5-minute resistance program to the hour-plus you've probably spent getting to and from the gym, changing, driving, etc. No wonder the resolution to work out regularly so often falls by the wayside after an initial bout of enthusiasm. According to the Centers for Disease Control and Prevention, only 19 percent of women do resistance exercise two or more times a week. And honestly, how often do you actually make it to the gym? On the other hand, anyone can find 5 minutes a day. It's less time than you probably take to shower, brush and floss your teeth, read your kid a bedtime story, empty the dishwasher, fold the laundry, or pay a few bills. Somehow you find the time to do these essential activities. Your fitness and weight-control program is equally important to your well-being.

TARGETING KEY MUSCLE GROUPS

The human body has more than 640 muscles. Do we need to work them all? Even traditional exercise can't hit them all. Ideally, there are 12 muscle groups you should train in a resistance program. We need to focus on these from an aesthetic, metabolic, and general health perspective. We'll omit directly isolating certain muscles such as the trapezius, forearm (extensors and flexors), and calves. Let me explain why. First, these muscles get worked *indirectly* through other activities and exercises. Second, over-strengthening these muscles can actually lead to postural issues, functional issues, and possibly injury.

The only other muscle groups I don't address in the resistance exercises that you'll be doing are the pectorals (chest) muscles. In my Los Angeles studio, I rarely (if ever) give women pec exercises, whether pushups, chest presses, or flys, because they can curve your posture forward, as we discussed earlier, actually making you look shorter and stouter. Men can introduce some chest exercises after the first month, or later on if you want to

Sets and Reps

Each time you perform an exercise or lift a weight, it is considered a repetition, or a rep for short. Each group of reps constitutes a set. The more reps in a set, the fewer sets you'll need to fatigue the muscle(s) involved.

expand the program. Unless you have access to a cable resistance machine or you're in the 1 percent of the population who can do more than 10 pullups, training your lat muscles will pose a challenge, so we'll omit them for now. As you become more advanced, I suggest you add them to your regular resistance program. Another muscle group, the adductors (inner thigh), can be worked indirectly through various lunge movements, which are adequate for beginners and intermediates. As you become more advanced, it's a good idea to find a place to use a cable resistance machine to isolate your inner thighs and add them to your program as well.

MUSCLE-BOUND? NO WAY!

I mentioned this concern at the start of the chapter, but I'd like to revisit it, since it's such a persistent misconception. Unfortunately, many people equate resistance exercise with bodybuilding. Women live in fear that it will make them big and bulky. Let's put that old wives' tale to rest. The fact is that there are three primary factors when it comes to getting bigger muscles, known as muscle hypertrophy. Number one is your hormonal status. Men get bigger muscles than women because we have more testosterone. It's as simple as that. Women who take testosterone, as some female bodybuilders do, get big muscles like men. But that is a deliberate strategy to increase their strength.

Second, if you want to build a bigger house, you need extra bricks and wood. If you just want to renovate your house and keep it the same size, it's very different from adding on an extension or a second story. It's the same thing with your body. Think of the bricks and wood as your food. You need to eat a lot of extra food to build new muscle tissue. As long as you're not taking testosterone and deliberately eating extra food, you're not going to get bigger.

There's one more factor, known as volume training, which is the opposite of the form of exercise I'm espousing in this book. Traditionally, bodybuilders strain to get bigger muscles. They'll select a specific body part, pick

Front and Back Muscles—
Plus Two Others

ANTERIOR	POSTERIOR
Pectorals (chest)	Rhomboids (upper back)
Anterior delts (shoulder)	Posterior delts (shoulder)
Biceps (front arm)	Triceps (back arm)
Rectus abs (front midsection)	Spinal erectors (lower back)
Quadriceps (front thigh)	Hamstrings (back thigh)
Transverse abs (corset) and Obliques (love handles)	

approximately four or five exercises per day for that body part, and then perform four or five sets of each exercise. That means that they're doing 16 to 25 sets for one specific body part each workout. That's what we call high-volume training.

Now that you understand the three key factors to make a muscle grow, you'll understand why if you don't take testosterone, don't deliberately supplement your diet to put on weight, and don't engage in high-volume training, your muscles aren't going to get bigger. They will, however, get denser, tighter, and stronger. Which is exactly what you want!

ONE EXERCISE A DAY, 5 MINUTES A DAY

Do the initial exercises in the order listed below:

1. Reverse Lunge

2. Superman

3. Lying Dumbbell Triceps Extension

4. Stiff-Leg Dumbbell Deadlift

5. Standing Dumbbell Curl Press

On the following 2 days, do these exercises:

1. Single-Arm Dumbbell Row

2. Standing Dumbbell Side Bend

The next week (Day 8), begin the cycle again.

You'll find complete instructions and photographs for all exercises starting on page 216.

ASSESS YOUR FITNESS LEVEL

I've provided three different approaches for each exercise, in ascending order of intensity. Base the number of repetitions you do on your current fitness level: Beginner, Intermediate, or Advanced. If you're a Beginner, you'll do 3 sets of 10 repetitions. If you're at an Intermediate level, you'll do 3 sets of 20 reps. And if you're Advanced, you'll do 3 sets of 30 reps. Once you identify your level of fitness, you'll follow the prescribed regimen of number of sets and reps. Obviously, if you overestimate initially, simply drop back a level.

Remember, the object of resistance exercise is to stress the muscle fibers so that they heal stronger, meaning you need to push yourself. You should barely be able to get to the prescribed number of repetitions, with perfect technique and minimal pausing. If you're unable to complete the prescribed number of repetitions or your technique is compromised, go lighter on the weights or do fewer repetitions. If you're not used to using weights, perhaps you'll need to cut back on the reps. Initially, I advise you to worry less about

Opposing Muscles

To maintain anterior (front) and posterior (back) muscles and optimal posture, it's important to work both the extensor muscles, in which the connected bones move apart when the muscle is contracted, as in a triceps extension, and the flexor muscles, in which the connected bones move closer together when the muscle contracts, as in a biceps curl.

the amount of resistance (the weights you'll use for several of the exercises) than about being able to handle the repetitions. So it's better to do 3 sets of 10 reps as a beginner using 3-pound weights than to use 5-pound weights and not be able to complete all the sets. On the other hand, if you're finding some exercises too easy, feel free to use a heavier set of weights to make it more challenging.

If you're new to resistance exercise, start at the Beginner level until you feel confident and strong enough to move on. If you're accustomed to this kind of workout, you may well be at the Intermediate level. If you're already quite strong and used to resistance exercise, you may be able to start at the Advanced level. It's always better to begin at a lower level, gain competence and confidence, and then move up. Find a level of exertion that feels comfortable (but not *too* comfortable) for you.

START WITH A WARMUP

A warmup can be useful before any sort of resistance exercise. My advice is to march (raise your knees as high as you can) or jog in place for 30 seconds, followed by 30 seconds of jumping jacks, before beginning your resistance exercise of the day. After only 5 minutes of exercise, there's no need to worry about a cooldown period. Between each set of exercises, you'll also rest for 60 seconds. Regardless of fitness level, you'll have 1 minute of warmup and 1 minute of rest between sets.

The 5 minutes refers to the time you're actually performing the exercise; however, rather than watch the clock or set a timer, simply complete the number of sets and reps appropriate for your fitness level. Depending on whether you're at the Beginner, Intermediate, or Advanced level and how quickly you perform each exercise, the elapsed time will differ. Obviously, doing a total of 30 reps will not take as long as doing 90. If you're a Beginner, it will actually take you less than 5 minutes to do a total of 30 reps. If you're at the Intermediate level, you're looking at 5 or 6 minutes to do 60 reps. If you're Advanced, it might take up to 7 minutes to do a total of 90 reps.

In the next chapter, we'll discuss the third component of My 5, which complements resistance exercise: aerobic activity in general and, specifically, taking 10,000 steps a day, every day!

Five Key Points in Chapter 2

1. Both structured/contrived exercise and overall movement are important for weight control, but we overrate the former and underrate the latter. Instead, flip that ratio by making a point of moving as much as possible throughout the day, as well as engaging in resistance exercise.

2. Resistance exercise refers to a muscle or muscle group working against a certain resistance (your own body weight or a the weight of dumbbell, for example) for a short period of time until it's fatigued. In contrast, aerobic exercise includes walking or anything that raises your heart rate, and is limited by general fatigue. Resistance exercise and aerobic activity are two pillars of My 5.

3. Resistance exercise helps rev up your metabolism so you burn more calories at rest, offsets your tendency to burn fewer calories as you slim down, protects lean muscle mass, prompts the release of hormones that help build muscle, and burns fat, shaping and sculpting your body so you look leaner, among numerous other benefits. Resistance exercise helps you avoid weight gain and, in concert with diet and the other behavior changes inherent in My 5, aids weight loss.

4. Resistance exercise doesn't require long workouts in a gym on fancy machines. Based on the latest research, my revolutionary approach maximizes intensity and minimizes time. You can do it for a mere 5 minutes in your home, working one muscle group a day, in a moderately intense manner. The key is consistency, meaning you'll do it every day.

5. The My 5 resistance exercise program is adaptable to every level of fitness, from Beginner to Advanced, and is designed to allow you to make modifications and add variety as you build your strength and endurance in a number of ways. Specific exercises with photos and instructions start on page 216.

CHAPTER

WALK IT OFF

As a teenager I was obsessed with bodybuilding, a passion that continued though my college and grad school years, during which I also worked as a fitness trainer. Every month I would read *Muscle and Fitness, MuscleMag, Flex,* and *Muscle Media 2000* cover to cover. Armed with the latest and greatest muscle-building routines I found in the magazines, I would spend nearly 2 hours a day in the gym lifting heavy weights, set after set, until I could barely walk. After years of studying exercises science and experimenting on myself, plus working with thousands of clients, my thinking has evolved. As I've explained, I've come to the conclusion that as a culture, we both overexercise and are underactive because we've created this artificial divide between the routine activities of daily life and the deliberate, intensive movements that we call "exercise." And we've been mistakenly valuing the latter over the former. This chapter is all about movement, as measured by the number of steps you take each day—the third component of My 5. Let me explain.

Imagine a woman—let's call her Jane—who's typical of many of my clients. She drives her car or takes the train to work, sitting for an hour. She then spends 8 hours at her desk, either heading out for lunch only to sit down in a coffee shop or eating at her desk. At the end of the workday, Jane logs another hour of sitting on her return trip in the car or on the train. When she gets home, she pops something in the microwave, sits down to eat, and then plops down in front of the TV or her computer. During a 24-hour period, Jane's spent almost all her waking hours seated.

Okay, you may be thinking. Well, I sit a good deal of the day, but I also get to the gym several days a week, and when I'm there, I work my tail off. So let's imagine a different scenario for Jane. Her workday and mode of travel remain the same, but she stops on her way home to take an hour-long spin class. After a vigorous workout, Jane is ravenous. So she picks up a fresh-pressed juice, which contains about 450 calories, to hold her over until dinner. She has a reservation at a nearby restaurant, but rather than walk there, she says to herself, "You know what, I just did the spin class and I'm pretty wiped. I'll drive there." Jane meets her friend, and after dinner, when the dessert menu appears, she confides, "After that spin class I did earlier, I deserve a little dessert."

Do you see where I'm going?

In the second scenario, Jane has indeed exercised, but she's been inactive for the rest of the day. Nor has she made any progress in expending more energy than she's consumed. Now let's look at how you can become a moving object. The third component of the My 5 Plan is taking 10,000 steps a day. This chapter isn't just about walking, although of course walking is integral to movement. Before we get into the details of this, let's do a little time travel.

THE GOOD OLD DAYS

Our great-grandparents did laundry by rubbing it on a washboard or putting it through a wringer washer and then hanging it out to dry. Kids would indeed walk miles to and from school. When Mrs. Jones needed to borrow a

cup of flour from Mrs. Smith, she'd walk over to get it. Most likely, your for-
bears earned their living with some sort of manual labor. Many people lived
on farms, toiling in the fields or barn from dawn to dusk. They grew food in
their gardens, digging, plowing, raking, weeding, and harvesting by hand.
Then they'd can, preserve, dehydrate, or pickle the harvest. The routines of
daily life demanded almost constant physical effort throughout the day.

Contrast that way of life with what is now the norm for most of us. Our
jobs often involve sitting at a desk. We buy our fruit and vegetables at a
supermarket or farm stand or order online from FreshDirect. We toss our
dirty clothes in the washing machine and then transfer them to the dryer.
The dishwasher takes care of dirty dishes and cutlery. We hop in the car,
even for short trips. And then there are the television, the computer, and all
the other digital toys we love so much. Yes, they entertain us and even stimulate our brains, but not so our muscles.

The group known as the Old Order Amish has opted to avoid modern
conveniences such as automobiles and electric appliances. They live much as
many of our forebears did, with most making their living as farmers or trades-
people. This lifestyle, so different from the sedentary life most North Americans live, makes them a valuable subject of scientific research on activity,
metabolism, and health. In a study of almost 100 Amish adults, subjects wore
an electronic monitor for a week and kept detailed logs of their activities.[1] In
that week, the Amish men spent 43 hours engaged in moderate activity,
10 hours in vigorous activity, plus 12 hours walking. On average, they took
18,500 steps a day, about 9 miles, resting only on Sunday. In comparison, their
wives, sisters, and daughters were relatively "lazy," walking only 5.7 hours each
week! Guess what? Only a quarter of the men and 27 percent of the women
were overweight; none of the men and only 9 percent of the women were obese.

Compare that to the statistics for all Americans: More than two-thirds of
adults are overweight and, according to the Centers for Disease Control and
Prevention, 35.7 percent of them are obese. The typical person takes about
5,100 steps a day, with men walking more than women.[2] With an obesity rate
of only 8 percent and 3 percent, respectively, Switzerland and Japan put us to

shame.[3,4] People in those countries regularly take close to 10,000 steps a day,[5,6] the minimum to which healthy adults should strive.[7]

THE DOWNSIDE OF TECHNOLOGY

Other than the Amish and a few other sects, I don't know of anyone who's willing to give up all these modern conveniences altogether, but there's no question that we pay a price for relying on them. We pay with compromised health, lack of energy, excess pounds, and slack muscles. We've become victims of our own "good" life. Why go Christmas shopping at the mall when you can just go to amazon.com? Everything—from your kid's diapers to 3-dozen rolls of toilet paper to exotic flowers just flown in from Colombia—is just a click away. And it's the same thing with socialization. There's no need to get together in person when you can Skype night and day. In Chapter 5, we'll talk about how linking to others via your electronic devices rather than in face-to-face encounters is just as unhealthy for your mental and physical health as not being active.

Don't worry. I'm not suggesting that we return to the early 20th century. There's a simple solution right at hand—or I should say foot? We already engage in one form of physical activity without even thinking about it. (We even dub our infants "toddlers" once they master the skill.) I'm talking about walking, of course. This perfectly natural human behavior is also a great way to help stay fit and slim. But let's take a step backward and speak first about movement in general.

GET A MOVE ON

Your objective is to increase the amount of what we fitness experts call chronic submaximal movement—translation: regular, frequent, and moderate intensity activity—throughout the day. Scientists refer to it as non-exercise activity thermogenesis, or NEAT for short, meaning the energy we burn while brushing our teeth, making meals, transferring clothes from the washer to the dryer, or vacuuming. NEAT activities are the ones we do every day

Why You Want to Move (Not Too Fast) All Day

Numerous studies show that regular moderate aerobic exercise raises your metabolism and improves the likelihood of preventing weight regain after losing pounds.[8, 9] It also has numerous other health benefits:

1. Reducing fat mass, which helps build and preserve muscle mass[10]

2. Strengthening your heart and lungs[11, 12]

3. Improving your cholesterol and triglyceride indicators[13, 14]

4. Protecting your bones and preventing bone loss[15, 16]

5. Improving insulin and blood sugar control, which deflects diabetes[17, 18]

6. Reducing blood pressure levels[19, 20]

7. Improving your mood and reducing stress[21]

8. Improving your sleep[22]

9. Minimizing the pain from arthritis[23]

10. Reducing the incidence of colds, flu, and other virus-borne illnesses[24, 25]

without going near a gym. Although we don't regard them as "exercise," they play a huge role in burning calories. And you're going to become more conscious of them and their importance in losing those pesky 5 pounds.

We've discussed changing your eating habits and spending about 5 minutes a day doing resistance exercise. In this chapter, we'll focus on aerobic activity. (You may want to review "The Other Kind of Exercise" for how aerobic activity differs from resistance exercise on page 34.) Any activity that makes you breathe harder is aerobic in nature. Some forms of activity, such as stair climbing and walking uphill, combine aerobic and resistance exercise.

Your goal is to become a body in motion. If that brings to mind images of a kung fu master leaping into the air and performing amazing feats, fear not. Rather, I want you to become a person who consciously engages in activity indoors and out, whether climbing stairs, doing household chores, or taking a walk with a friend. You'll be taking 10,000 steps a day—and more is even better.

Assuming your stride is close to the average of about 2½ feet—the longer your legs, the wider your stride—taking 10,000 steps is roughly the equivalent of walking 5 miles. You can keep track of it either way. I know, 10,000 steps may sound huge, but you'll be pleasantly surprised how quickly they add up.

MAKE TRACKS

Before we go any further, let me reiterate: being active is not just about walking; it's about moving. And when it comes to walking, here are a few tips:

- You don't need take those 10,000 steps in one sustained walk. In fact, I'd rather you didn't.

- You don't need to walk super fast, but you can if you like.

- You don't have to walk outside (although being outdoors in sunlight helps set your internal time clock, which, as you'll learn in Chapter 4, can play a role in weight loss).

I can almost hear some of you mumbling to yourselves, "How could I ever find the time to take 10,000 steps a day?" Remember, I'm not asking you to take one 5-mile walk each day. I *am* asking you to take 10,000 steps, as a way to tally your overall movement throughout the day. Being consistently active throughout the day is more beneficial than briskly walking 5 miles in one concentrated effort.

So, how do you rack up 10,000 steps and also have a life? The simple answer is that you'll incorporate them into your life with a few easy changes. (The more profound answer is that being active is an essential part of your life, not an afterthought.) If you're already reasonably active, running after small children all day or walking your dog a few times a day, for example, you might be surprised to find that you're already putting in close to 2 miles a day. So the goal of 10,000 steps may not be that much of a reach for you. And guess what? Walking can be enjoyable. And research shows that you're more likely to stick with a moderate and fun approach rather than a vigorous exercise program.[26]

On the other hand, if you're currently a bona fide couch potato, logging 10,000 steps a day will be more of a challenge, but it is perfectly achievable, as I'll show you. First, though, let me triage the strategy:

- Far and away the most important thing is to keep moving throughout the day. Try being slightly "less efficient," such as parking your car farther away from an entry.

- "Formal" walks, whether around the block or longer distances, are part of that process, but hardly the whole enchilada.

- Finally, achieving a good pace when you take walks maximizes the aerobic benefits, but don't worry about that if you're new to walking for fitness.

My advice is to never be still, except when you're sleeping, eating, or traveling in a car, train, or plane.

PUTTING IT ALL TOGETHER

There's overwhelming evidence that people who walk more tend to be slimmer than those who walk less.[27-32] Did you know that obese people on average sit for $2\frac{1}{2}$ hours more each day than lean people? And that lean people stand and walk an average of more than 2 additional hours a day than obese people?[33] Again, it's also more effective to be in motion throughout the day than to be inactive for 23 hours and then engage in 1 hour of exercise.[34] Likewise, regular moderate activity is more effective than being a couch potato all day and then taking a grueling run before retreating to the couch.[35]

Most people find it easier to take two or more shorter walks throughout the day, in addition to NEAT activity. Fit those walks into your regular schedule, whenever you want to take a break at the office, for instance, or pick up the mail, walk the dog, or hand out flyers for a neighborhood get-together. In a sense, the object is to make your life a little *less* efficient. Yes, you read that right!

DO AS I DO

Here's how I make my life a little *less* efficient. When I'm not traveling, I follow a certain pattern. After I wake up, I walk to the coffee shop near my house to get my caffeine fix. Yes, I could make coffee at home, and I used to do that, but the truth is that walking there and back takes 3,200 steps, meaning I'm almost one-third of the way to reaching my 10,000 steps. And what a great way to start the day! I do the same thing later for my work break. Those 6,400 daily steps translate to about 3 miles. Over the course of a year, the caloric expenditure of walking to and from the coffee shop twice a day every day burns enough calories to lose 20 or 30 pounds a year, all without changing anything else in my life.

So, is having a coffee machine at home actually efficient, or is that inefficient when I look at my total life? How much time would I have to spend in the gym if I were making coffee at home and therefore not walking to the coffee shop? Now, I'm not telling you to make a coffee run twice a day—or even to drink coffee. I'm using it as an example of ways to change our daily habits to burn more calories without necessarily taking any additional time. Feel free to make your coffee at home, if you prefer, and find other ways to get your steps in.

I also try to make my lunch meetings within walking distance of my office. I have an earpiece on my cellphone, and when I have calls to make, I

Five (Plus Two) Ways to Be *Less* Efficient

1. Park your car at the far end of the lot.

2. Take the stairs instead of the elevator or escalator.

3. Make lunch dates at places within walking distance of your workplace.

4. Walk the kids to the school bus stop instead of driving them.

5. Get off the bus 5 or 10 blocks from your office or other destination.

6. Walk up and down each aisle in the supermarket, even if you are not buying anything in that aisle.

7. In an airport terminal, bypass the moving platform.

Find Your Bliss

While I'm a great fan of walking, plenty of other forms of moderate-intensity aerobic activities will provide many of the same benefits. I've recently taken up golf. Did you know that walking a typical 18-hole golf course takes more than 10,000 steps?[39] (Don't you dare use a golf cart!) I actually clock about 14,000 steps on my Fitbit. You just propel yourself forward. Other great forms of aerobic exercise you may already be enjoying include swimming, bicycling on a level surface, doubles tennis, gardening, slow dancing, Zumba, in-line skating, water aerobics, and ice skating.

walk. I'll either pace inside or walk slowly around the block. Within reason, whenever I'm in an office building, I take the stairs.

You want to get in the mind-set of moving from the moment you wake up until the moment you go to bed. I try to get my clients to do the same. "Look, unless you're eating or traveling in a car or a train or a plane," I say to them, "don't sit." My staff and I all have standing desks at the office. Since we made this switch, we have had fewer sick days and fewer problems with lower back pain. Standing and leaning forward supported by a desk reduces muscle tension in the lower back and hips.[36] This is hardly a new idea. Thomas Jefferson, Charles Darwin, and Ernest Hemingway all worked at standing desks, so you'll be in good company if you decide to do the same. You also burn more calories standing at a desk than you do sitting at one.[37] Then there's a walking desk—you may have heard of this latest spin on a standing desk. For the ultimate multitasker, a walking desk combines a desk with a treadmill in place of a chair. Walking 1 mile per hour on the treadmill burns about one-third more calories than sitting at a conventional desk.[38] There's even a bicycle desk in the works.

INTEGRATE ACTIVITY INTO YOUR SOCIAL LIFE

Even if you live in an area without numerous opportunities to engage in outdoor activities, you can always find a park or nature center to walk in and urban neighborhoods to explore. Instead of joining your buddies for dinner and a film—you'll be sitting on your derriere for hours—why not suggest a walk followed by dinner? How about packing a picnic lunch and taking a hike with another family? Rather than sitting at a coffee shop, why not get your latte to go and take a short walk with a pal or work friend? Not only is it more intimate than sitting surrounded by strangers, but walking together also opens up possibilities such as exploring a newly opened store. Get in the habit of taking a walk after dinner with your partner. If you're a new mother feeling housebound and lonely, put your babe in the stroller and head off to the nearest playground. You're almost guaranteed to run into other moms.

I'll often meet a friend for a hike. We walk, socialize, and enjoy the fresh air and scenery. What's not to like? Recently, I was playing golf with a new client. After telling me that he played four days a week, he said, "It's tough to get to the gym on those days to get in my cardio on the treadmill." I replied that there was no need to get on the treadmill if he was playing 18 holes of golf, which provides 50 percent more cardio benefit than anything else he could be doing at the gym. More good news: Research shows that people who participate with friends or family in a weight-loss program are more likely to stay on track and to maintain their new weight.[40]

MOVEMENT INHIBITORS

So why do so many of us move as little as possible? We may not deliberately avoid using our legs to get from here to there, but nonetheless, out of habit or because our suburban neighborhood has no sidewalks, we often don't take full advantage of this wonderful form of aerobic exercise. Or perhaps we simply live too far from stores, schools, parks, playgrounds, and other destinations for it to be practical to walk. No wonder city dwellers, who live closer to such amenities, are healthier and tend to have a longer life expectancy than people who live in suburban (and even rural) locales and rely on cars.[41, 42] For every additional hour spent in a car each day, people are on average 6 percent *more* likely to be obese, and conversely, almost 5 percent *less* likely to be obese for each additional kilometer (⅝ mile) they walk per day.[43] A British study found that people who walk to work were 45 percent more physically active during the workweek than those who drove to work, and the walkers engaged in 60 percent more moderate to vigorous physical activity.[44]

Men's Health magazine conducts an annual study to find out which American cities have the fittest population, meaning the lowest rates of obesity. Leading the list is Boulder, Colorado, with an obesity rate of only 12.5 percent. Guess what? Among 14 cities of similar size, Boulder has the highest number of people who walk to work, and is second among those who ride their bicycles to work. What's called "active transportation" is associated with lower rates of obesity.[45]

Other "fit" towns, including Charlottesville, Virginia; Bellingham, Washington; and Fort Collins–Loveland, Colorado, are blessed with a multitude of state and local parks, national forests, trails, running paths, and amenities that provide the opportunities to walk, cycle, swim, ski, hike, and engage in numerous other outdoor activities. These towns actually have a culture that values getting outdoors and moving about. Cities with access to good public transportation, such as Colorado Springs, Denver, and Portland, Oregon, also tend to have a higher proportion of fit people.[46, 47]

THE USA IS OUT OF STEP

Several years ago, I took off nearly a year from my practice and traveled to the 10 healthiest countries in the world (mainly determined by average life expectancy and inversely related to obesity) to study what their residents eat and how they burn those calories. Big surprise: There was no common denominator in terms of diet. In one country, dairy played a large role in the diet; in another country, no one ate dairy. In one country, people ate with chopsticks; elsewhere, they used forks. And so on. The only common denominator in all 10 countries: Their populations all walk more than we do in the United States. Canada, my homeland, came in at a respectable number 8, but, sad to say, the United States didn't even make the top 50.

The Serious Consequences of Sitting

Our default activity (or more properly, inactivity) these days is sitting, all too often in front of the television or computer. Not surprisingly, spending too much time on your behind is associated with obesity.[49, 50] Sitting is also an independent risk factor for chronic disease.[51–53] That means that excessive sitting itself, not just the absence of aerobic activity, is risky behavior. Study after study links sitting with an increased risk of heart disease and cancer. Sitting for long periods of time is actually worse for you than smoking.[54] According to Alberta Health Services–Cancer Care in Canada, too much time in the car or in a chair results in almost 160,000 cases of cancer annually, a third again as many as those caused by smoking.[55] One study reveals that for every hour you spend on your behind, you shorten your life span by an average of 22 minutes.[56] That's slightly more than 1 hour for every 3 hours seated!

The average American walks 5,117 steps a day, whereas someone in Switzerland walks an average of 9,650 steps a day, almost twice as much.[48] So right off the bat, regardless of genetic predisposition to certain diseases, regardless of dietary intake or daily calorie consumption, someone who walks about 5 miles a day is going to be slimmer, healthier, and live longer than a person who walks half that much. Fact! RealAge.com, which assesses your "real" age in terms of how you feel, claims that taking 10,000 steps a day is the equivalent of subtracting about 4½ years from your chronological age for women and about 4 years for men.

WHAT WALKING CAN (AND CANNOT) DO

Moderate exercise of any sort *on its own* probably won't help you shed pounds. But in concert with dietary and other lifestyle changes—that's what My 5 is all about—walking can help you achieve and maintain weight loss. Walking at a brisk pace burns 3 to 4 more calories a minute than you'd burn if you were quietly sitting in a chair. I know that doesn't sound like a lot, but considering that there are 960 waking minutes a day, we're talking of a difference in the thousands of calories! In one 6-month study, over-weight sedentary women were divided into two groups. Women in one group cut back on the total number of calories they ate by 25 percent. Meanwhile, the other group cut calorie intake by only 12.5 percent but exercised 12.5 percent more than the first group.[57] Both groups created the same calorie deficit, 25 percent, and all the women lost about a pound of weight per week. Here's the takeaway: It wasn't the walking *per se* that resulted in modest weight loss. It was the calorie deficit itself.

Let me put aside one another misconception. Walking can be of enormous value in forestalling weight gain. Once you've lost the 5 pounds I've promised you will on the My 5 Plan, you certainly don't want to regain it. A longitudinal study provides insight. It followed 5,000 young men and women over 15 years, during which most of them packed on more than 1 pound a year, which is a fairly standard rate. However, individuals who regularly walked more than 15 minutes a day gained significantly less weight, and some gained none.[58] We lose muscle mass and our hormones change as we age, but these effects are compounded by sedentary behavior. The good news it that we can stall some of the effects of aging with a regular walking program, as well as with resistance exercise.

DO YOU HAVE TO DO YOUR WALKING ALL AT ONCE?

According to the updated recommendations for adults from the American College of Sports Medicine and the American Heart Association, the answer is no.[59] All that matters is the accumulation of activity. This is great news for those of you who need to squeeze in your aerobic activity here and there throughout the day. Taking several shorter walks may be more appealing—or less intimidating—and also provide a psychological benefit. In one study, a group of overweight and previously sedentary women was instructed to take a daily 30-minute walk; another group was assigned three 10-minute walks throughout the day. At the end of the study, the researchers found that

Five More Ways to Make the Steps Add Up

1. Make more food and beverage destinations within walking distance.

2. If you must drive to a restaurant, forget the valet parking. Instead, park a block or more away. It helps your digestion to move around after sitting down to eat.

3. Join a walking group or a hiking club.

4. Check out social media groups and similar websites to find hikes, walking (or stair-climbing) fundraisers, and other active events near you.

5. During those endless TV ads, hop up and use that time to change the sheets, wipe down the kitchen counter, or empty the trash.

the women in the second group were more self-motivated and more likely to continue their walking regimen in the future.[60] Again, these were previously sedentary people.

PACE YOURSELF

Now that you know how all the everyday things that keep you moving are part of your weight-control program, let's talk a bit more about walking, as in taking a walk. Am I asking you to power-walk or walk at a certain pace? Absolutely not, but rather than just strolling aimlessly along, you do want to walk as though you had a destination in mind—what I call walking with intention. Don't get hung up on being the speediest strider in the neighborhood; on the other hand, you don't want to be the slowest one either! Instead, think of yourself as someone with things to do and places to go.

If you're used to running, jogging, or even sprinting, feel free to log some of your miles that way if you wish, but there's no need to do so. Jogging or fast running burns more calories than walking does because you're projecting your body up as well as forward. Again, do what works for you at a comfortable pace. Rather than worry about your rate of perceived exertion, know that as long as you can walk at a brisk pace and carry on a conversation without gasping for breath, you're not overdoing it. Over time, your pace may well increase as you slim down and develop more muscle mass (as we'll discuss in Chapter 7).

WHAT'S ENOUGH?

The greatest benefit from exercise, at least in terms of extending life span, occurs in the first 20 minutes. If you follow the current Centers for Disease Control and Prevention guidelines of 150 minutes of moderate aerobic exercise a week, plus muscle-strengthening activities two or more times a week,[63] you'll cut your risk of premature death from any cause by almost 20 percent.[64] But triple that amount of exercise in a week and the mortality risk decreased by only an additional 4 percent. Not that any extra time isn't desirable, but the point is that the initial effort brings the largest reward. That's powerful motivation to get moving.

But can you exercise too much? In one study, 400 middle-age women were divided into three groups and told to maintain their customary way of eating

5 Five Aids to Help You Move (More)

Whether you're out early on a July morning or late on a January afternoon, dress in layers of clothing, so you can shed one as you warm up. Some motivators to get you moving include:

1. A pedometer/activity monitor. Wear it not just on walks but also from the time you get up until you turn off the light. For more, see page 69.

2. Comfortable walking shoes (see "Happy Feet" on page 70) and socks that cushion your feet and wick away moisture.

3. Music to walk by.

4. A walking partner. If someone's waiting for you on the corner, you'd better be there!

5. A journal to track your activity (see page 243).

How Walking Beats Running

Walking is a great low-impact alternative to running or jogging—it's easy on the hips and knees—with minimal risk of injury. (The reverse lunges that are part of your resistance exercise will strengthen the muscles that support those joints.) However, if you already like to jog or run, feel free. Just be sure that your joints are aligned and your leg muscles are strong enough to act as shock absorbers. Also, be sure to wear shoes that give you the right support. Both jogging and running will burn more calories than walking for the same length of time, but is there a long-term advantage?

When researchers at Lawrence Berkeley National Laboratory compared data on 33,000 runners and almost 16,000 walkers to ascertain the health benefits of each activity, walking had a slight overall edge.[62] Six years later, the researchers checked in on the study participants again. Both groups had reduced their blood pressure, total cholesterol, risk for cardiovascular disease, and risk for diabetes. But the walkers' improvements were better across the board, except for reduced diabetes risk, which was the same as it was for the runners. And the more the study subjects ran or walked, the greater the benefits. The only hitch is that walking obviously takes longer than running to see comparable results.

and work out at a gentle pace, such as walking or riding a stationary bike.[65] The first group was to exercise for 72 minutes a week, the second group for 136 minutes, and the third for 194 minutes. After 6 months, all the women had lost weight. The second group lost slightly more than first group, which did the least exercise. But surprisingly, the women in group three, who had done the most exercise, lost only half the amount of weight predicted, just slightly more than group one. Overall, there was no significant difference among the three groups' weight change. How come? Just like our imaginary friend Jane, the study subjects' extra exertions made their bodies fight back by increasing their appetite.

Your body has a mind of its own, thanks to its properties of homeostasis (the instinct to remain stable). Your body senses when you're in a state of serious calorie deficit—either as a result of starving yourself or overexercising—and adjusts accordingly, impacting a number of different hormones, which we'll discuss later in this chapter. As a result, your metabolism slows, which makes it harder to lose weight.

INTENSE EXERCISE CAN BACKFIRE

In a study in which the number of calories consumed by obesity-prone rats was slashed by 50 percent, they became less active and lost a little bit of weight.[65] But later, when the rats were allowed to eat as much as they wanted, they gained back even more weight than they'd lost. Humans are not unlike rats in this respect. A number of studies have shown that when obese sedentary subjects are put on an increased exercise program, some of them lose little or no weight. Despite the increased calorie expenditure, members of this subgroup compensated by eating more and being even more sedentary when they weren't performing the assigned exercise.[66]

There's a direct relationship between intense cardio activity and your appetite. Let's say that in her spin class, our old friend Jane burned about 200 calories. If she'd been sitting on the sofa, her resting metabolism would have burned about 180 calories. But that very same exercise stimulates an increase in appetite and food intake. And it's not just an immediate reaction. It persists over the next 12 to 24 hours. In other words, Jane might well end up consuming more calories than she has burned over the day. As a result of that structured, contrived form of physical activity (calories out), she felt she had "permission" to consume more treats (calories in). So the bottom line is that such intense, concentrated exercise actually runs the risk of making you less fit and more at risk for weight gain.

Women, Exercise, and Hormones

Women seem particularly subject to changes in the level of their appetite and energy-regulating hormones (ghrelin and insulin) after extensive exercise. Specifically, their appetite increases, their energy level decreases, and they're more likely to store fat. In one study, men displayed no real changes in these hormones, but women showed increased blood levels of ghrelin and decreased levels of insulin.[67] (For more on ghrelin and insulin and their role in weight gain, see page 81.) This phenomenon has created debate about whether women in particular shouldn't overexercise or create a calorie deficit from extreme dieting, because female bodies are more susceptible to fighting back in an effort to establish homeostasis than male bodies.

Pretty ironic, huh? I now know that there's a better approach, which I'll share with you in a moment, after we discuss another irony.

OVERDOING IT CAN INTERFERE WITH IMMUNITY

Another unintended consequence of overdoing exercise is stress on the immune system. Research suggests that moderate aerobic activity, such as walking, enhances immune response, while vigorous activity, such as running, may compromise it. One study found that mice that ran on tiny treadmills for 3 days until they were exhausted were more likely to get sick and to become seriously ill when exposed to a flu virus than mice that had simply rested in their cages.[68] But what would be the effect of moderate exercise?

Another group of researchers wondered the same thing. They infected mice with a virulent flu virus and divided them into three groups. Two of the groups ran on a treadmill during the initial stages of the flu before symptoms appeared.[69] The first group ran for hours until they were exhausted; the second group jogged slowly for 20 to 30 minutes; the third group rested. The process was repeated for 2 more days. The result? About 70 percent of the rats that ran until they were exhausted died. Half of the rats that just rested also died. But of the rats that jogged for only 20 to 30 minutes a day, only 18 percent succumbed. Moderate activity had stimulated their immune systems to fight the flu virus.

Pushing yourself to the point of exhaustion from exercise causes inflammation, which suppresses your immune system, making you far more vulnerable to the flu, other viruses, and illness in general.[70, 71] So, hey, forget about P90X and other extreme workout programs advertised on late-night TV. Instead, daily sessions of approximately 5 minutes of resistance exercise in combination with 10,000 daily steps will get you good results without the risks inherent in exercising too hard or too long.

STIMULATE YOUR BRAIN

Albert Einstein claimed that he came up with the theory of relativity while riding his bicycle. Our brains work better when we're in motion. I know mine certainly does. I've written most of my books while walking or cycling. Increased aerobic activity, alone or in combination with a weight-loss diet, leads to an improved sense of well-being[72] and enhanced sleep.[73] Physical activity brings more oxygen and blood to the brain. In one study that compared physically fit and less fit preteens, the fitter kids delivered better test results.[74] A study of more than a million Swedish 18-year-olds who enlisted in the military found that those who were more physically fit also had a higher IQ.[75]

Feeling blocked creatively? Get up and take a walk. In a series of studies, researchers at Stanford University found that simply walking outdoors upped the "divergent thinking" index of more than 80 percent of 176 college students, and walking on a treadmill raised it for 63 percent, in both cases compared with sitting.[76] The subjects were told to walk or sit for 4 minutes, during which they were asked to come up with alternative uses for a common object. Responses were considered creative if no one else came up with the same answer. Moreover, when tested again after returning to their desks, the students who had just walked found that

What Is Resting Metabolism?

Your metabolism never takes a break. You may be lying inert on your bed, or even be asleep, but your body is burning calories to power all its processes, from brain function to digestion. Your basal (resting) metabolism rate is the number of calories your body burns per hour at rest, which slows with age, hormonal changes, or weight gain. Your genes also come into play. Aerobic activity stokes your calorie-burning fire further, like turning your cooktop burner from low to medium or high. Your resting metabolism is the ground zero from which we measure the added caloric expenditure impact of any activity.

Which Burns More Calories: Running or Walking?

According to one of Sir Isaac Newton's laws of motion, moving the same weight over the same distance requires the same amount of energy. Therefore, the assumption was that someone running a mile burns the same number of calories as he or she would burn walking the same distance. However, running consumes more oxygen to power muscles than walking does, thus increasing the number of calories burned.[83] For example, if you weigh 145 pounds and walk 1 mile at a pace of 3 to 4 miles an hour, you'll burn about 44 calories over your resting metabolism. If you run that same mile, you'll burn about 91 calories over your resting metabolism.[84]

their inspirational juices continued to flow, compared with those who had been sitting all along.

Moderate (but not intense) exercise also improves memory. Just 30 minutes of moderate aerobic exercise before a test can improve memory and reduce the amount of time necessary to complete the test.[77] In a recent study, three groups of young German women listened to 30-minute recordings of nouns in their own language paired with the Polish equivalent. Two days later, they were tested on how well they remembered the Polish nouns.[78] Women in one group listened after simply sitting for half an hour, while the second group rode a stationary bike for half an hour before listening. Women in the third group, who rode the bicycles while listening to the recording, displayed significantly better recall than either of the other groups. The women who had been sedentary before listening remembered the fewest Polish words.

Walking has long been associated with a reduction in depression.[79] Walking a mere 30 minutes for 10 days can alleviate severe depression, according to one study.[80] How come? Walking stimulates endorphins, which are natural painkillers. A study in Scotland involving almost 20,000 men and women found that a mere 20 minutes a week (!) of any physical activity was all it took to avoid feeling "dour," or what we would call being in psychological distress.[81]

Walking in a natural environment or other quiet place can also be a form of stress-relieving meditation, as discussed in Chapter 5. Taking regular walks has also been shown to reduce cognitive decline in older people.[82] Regular walking can reduce stress and negative emotions, making you more able to maintain weight loss.

WALKING MINIMIZES THE RISK OF INJURY

In addition to increased appetite and the potential for weight gain, intense exercise can cause an array of injuries. Runners often experience twisted ankles, pulled tendons, shin splints, and a host of other problems. Of course, once a runner is sidelined, he or she cannot pursue that activity or others for a period of time. So overexercising can result in injury, which in turn leads to an underactive lifestyle, at least temporarily. Remember, it's the habitual, regular, ongoing moderate physical activity that keeps you slim, fit, and far less likely to suffer an injury

So here's the irony: By slowing down, you can actually reap the benefits of living an active lifestyle. Just understand that slowing down isn't at all the same thing as being inactive.

AN ACTIVITY MONITOR CAN MAKE YOU MORE ACTIVE

I've always encouraged my clients to find ways to keep moving throughout the day, advising them to take at least 10,000 steps a day, just as I'm doing with you. And I give them an activity monitor. Whatever brand you use, an activity monitor provides you with a gauge of how much you're moving. A basic pedometer counts the number of steps or miles you cover by sensing your body's movement and exertion level. Most also count the rough number of calories you burn, but they aren't

Happy Feet

The better your shoes fit, the more likely you are to walk and to enjoy it. The more you enjoy it, the more you'll stay on the move. Wear appropriate footgear. The high heels that make your legs look longer and slimmer may be fine for walking from your office to the conference room, but they're hardly suitable for long distances, uneven surfaces, or even climbing stairs. (Flats, flip-flops, and many sandals are just as problematic.) Needless to say, if your feet hurt, you're not going to be motivated to walk any farther than absolutely necessary. Keep a pair of comfortable shoes at the office for when you need to walk any distance.

Wearing high heels increases the incidence of knee and ankle injuries and may also aggravate or contribute to the development of bunions (as do poorly fitting shoes). For years I cared more about looking cool than having shoes that fit properly, and I paid the price by developing a painful tailor's bunion. Now I know better. In fact, for the past several years I've been designing New Balance cross-trainers for men and women. The idea is to have both maximum versatility and maximum comfort. My shoes are also super lightweight and should work equally well whether you're wearing jeans, playing tennis, or walking. Pick a shoe that's good-looking enough (as mine are!) so that you'll actually wear it, has enough room in the toe box, and supports your arches.

necessarily super accurate. The more data you can input into the monitor (gender, weight, height), the more accurate the number of calories burned is likely to be.

Some of the newer devices can even distinguish between a step and a stair, thanks to a built-in altimeter. A simple pedometer will set you back about $20, although there are lots of more elaborate products on the market. A pocket pedometer is about half the length of your thumb and can be clipped to your collar, waistband, bra, or other article of clothing, although it's a good idea to attach it to a security leash to avoid losing it. You can wear some monitors on your wrist. Manufacturers include Fitbit (my preference), Jawbone, Nike, and New Balance, among others. More advanced models, which cost about $60 and up, enable you to connect to a website or smartphone app to view data on your activity level, including when you're sedentary. Fitbit can provide graphs

on which day of the week you were most active, plus you can track your progress and compare it against your past performance and compete with friends.
New gadgets proliferate. Samsung and Apple both recently introduced a
watch that does double duty as an activity monitor and links to your smartphone. Some shoes even contain a pedometer now.

A number of studies confirm that the use of an activity monitor can result
in significantly increased activity.[85] One meta-study showed that people who
wore pedometers took, on average, more than 2,000 additional steps a day (an
almost 30 percent increase in physical activity) than individuals without
pedometers. Having a specific goal, such as 10,000 steps a day, boosts the likelihood of increased activity.[86, 87] In this respect, an activity monitor can be a
powerful motivator to change your behavior. Using a pedometer is associated
with a modest increase in weight loss[88] but a greater decrease in BMI.[89] Even if
you're not big on such metrics, just wearing a fitness monitor can be a silent
reminder to move more.

Five Places to Get In Your Steps

No place to walk safely outdoors or after dark? Try out these ideas to boost
the number of steps you take each day:

1. ON THE STAIRS. Walk up and down the stairs five times every few
hours. When you ascend the stairs, you're lifting your body weight up and
forward, combining weight-bearing and aerobic benefits.

2. ON THE PHONE. Pace while you chat or text.

3. IN THE FAMILY ROOM. Do side steps (left foot to the right and
back, right foot to left and back, and so on) as you fold laundry or watch
television.

4. IN THE BATHROOM. Walk in place while brushing your teeth or your
hair.

5. AT THE CLOSEST MALL. Most welcome walkers before the stores
open.

THE FALLBACK OPTION

Let's return to my initial distinction between "exercise" and frequent, regular movement. Even if you walk 10,000 steps in one sustained effort, perhaps an hour and a half on a treadmill at the gym after sitting all day, it's not the same as moving enough throughout the day to log the same number of steps. I also prefer moving outside if at all possible. That said, if all you can fit into your day is one long walk, that's all you can do.

The same applies to using machines at a gym. I'm in favor of anything that engages you in physical activity, whether it's an Arc Trainer, a Helix Lateral Trainer, an elliptical trainer, or a treadmill. Sometimes, getting 10,000 steps in throughout the day is impossible, and we need to supplement our daily routine with a cardio machine. On days when I'm flying for 12 or 14 hours, I have no choice. When I finally get to my hotel, I'll return e-mails and phone calls while using the Arc Trainer or elliptical trainer. Cardio exercise machines are useful tools to supplement activity. But not everybody has access to a gym, and not everyone needs a gym. I want people to get away from this notion that exercise is something that has to be planned out and done in a specific building at a specific time on a specific piece of equipment. Still, the bottom line is that I just want people to move more.

Five Ways to Walk Safely

If you must walk on the street and/or at night, be sure to follow these guidelines:

1. Walk facing the oncoming traffic.

2. Wear light-colored clothing after dark.

3. Wear reflective clothes and shoes and carry a flashlight or attach a flashing reflector to your clothing after dark.

4. Avoid walking at dusk, when visibility is poor.

5. Carry a cellphone in case you need to call for help.

Five Key Points in Chapter 3

1. Our sedentary lifestyle plays a major role in the epidemic of obesity in the United States, despite an obsession with dieting and exercise. Intense exercise can actually increase appetite and (mistakenly) justify overeating, negating any calorie-burning benefit. Instead, you want to sit as little as possible and be in motion throughout the day.

2. Regular moderate aerobic exercise raises your metabolism, helping reduce the likelihood of regaining lost pounds. It also improves insulin and blood sugar control so you're less likely to store fat, improves your sleep (which independently helps control weight), and helps build or preserve muscle mass, which tones your body. And it does so without significantly increasing your appetite.

3. Using a pedometer or other monitoring device to track your movement throughout the day allows you to quantify your movement and can be a motivational tool. Your objective is to take a minimum of 10,000 steps a day, the equivalent of about 5 miles.

4. Becoming aware of how we depend on driving (sitting) or public trans-portation (usually sitting) for short trips can lead to behavior changes that enhance weight-loss efforts. For instance, it may actually take twice as long to get in an hour's workout if you drive to a gym and back rather than just head out the door for a walk.

5. Copious research links more steps walked on a regular basis to lower weight, greater ability to keep lost pounds from returning, improved health, and increased longevity.

I've cited a number of research studies in this chapter and would like to close with one that sums up the idea that the greatest benefit of moderate exercise, such as taking 10,000 steps a day, comes from doing it every single day of your life. That's why seeing exercise as an event-based activity—going to the gym three times a week, for example—won't get you the results you want. In a long-term study that followed more than 34,000 women, the subjects reported on their weight and activity level seven times from 1992 to 2007. They gained an average of 6 pounds over the years, but a small group of them gained virtually none. Those women engaged in moderate exercise, comparable to brisk waking, for about an hour every day.[90] The study authors concluded that the consistency with which the women exercised made the difference in their ability to maintain their weight, as opposed to the other women, who all gained weight over the years. Remember two words regarding aerobic activity: *moderate* and *consistent,* as in every day!

Now read on to learn how getting enough sleep will help you bid goodbye to 5 pounds in as many days, by following the My 5 Plan.

CHAPTER

4

SNOOZE TO LOSE

I've always tried to get close to 8 hours of sleep a night and have been aware of the importance of sleep from an early age. When I'm sleep deprived, my cravings—particularly for sugar—rule my food choices. My wife jokes that for every hour less than 8 hours of sleep I get, I tend to eat an extra chocolate chip cookie the next day! When I'm overtired, I don't feel like exercising either. It's almost dangerous for me to do so. But when I'm well rested, I find it easy to eat proactively and am full of energy to keep moving.

No one disputes that you can lose weight by eating less (at least short-term), especially in tandem with regular physical activity. But does the amount of shut-eye you get every night *really* have any bearing on your weight? Until recently, addressing insufficient sleep was the neglected component of weight loss. However, there's now a considerable body of research that unquestionably links the two.

According to David Klein, MD, one of the leading sleep physicians in North America, instead of taking an hour off from work to go to lunch or the gym, people might be better off taking a 30-minute power nap. His suggestion made me rethink the importance of sleep in a way that I never had before. Take vitamin supplementation as analogy. I'm not a big believer in vitamin supplements. If someone is already getting all the micronutrients needed through diet, additional vitamins and minerals most likely won't help at all. But for those who are deficient in a certain micronutrient, the addition of a daily multivitamin could be life changing. Likewise, if you're not getting enough sleep, an additional 30 minutes a day could literally transform your body and overall health.

I'm seeing a definite shift in the thinking about sleep. People used to boast about how little sleep they needed. Today, even highly competitive types, whether CEOs or athletes, seem to understand how essential it is to spend at least 7 hours in the sack in order to perform at the top of their game. An article on the Huffington Post drove this point home with quotes from such movers and shakers as Sheryl Sandberg, Jennifer Lopez, Ellen DeGeneres, the Dalai Lama, and Warren Buffett on how important sleep is to them.[1]

In the introduction to her recent book *Thrive,* Arianna Huffington talks about the wakeup call she received when she collapsed from burnout and exhaustion several years ago. After leading a high-paced life and sleeping only 4 or 5 hours a night, she made some serious lifestyle changes and now aims for 7 to 8 hours a night. She declares that getting enough sleep is the key to being successful, recommending (tongue-in-cheek) that women literally "sleep their way to the top."[2]

When I start working with a new client, I'll ask him or her to e-mail me each night yes or no responses to the five questions on which My 5 is based. Without fail, the most common behavior people fail to achieve is getting adequate sleep. Recently, I was asked to speak at a conference in San Diego. I had all 800 attendees anonymously participate in a questionnaire that asked them which of the five behaviors they'd fulfilled over the past 24 hours. A staggering 86 percent replied no to the question "Did you sleep at least 7 hours last night?"

If you're getting less than 7 (or better yet, 8) hours of sleep a night, your weight-loss efforts could be significantly hampered. Sleep-deprived people have been shown to eat more, and particularly to eat more refined carbohydrates, which can contribute to weight gain, as we discussed in Chapter 1.[3] Likewise, if the *quality* of your sleep is compromised, you may find it difficult to lose weight. Along with a good diet and enough exercise, getting a good night's rest is integral to overall good health and a sense of well-being, but sleep duration and quality also have a specific impact on weight.

ENEMIES OF SLEEP

Our contemporary lifestyle is incompatible with good sleeping habits on multiple levels. Some changes in our lifestyle occurred more than a century ago; others are more recent. A large 1960 survey found that people averaged between 8 and almost 9 hours of sleep a night.[4] National Sleep Foundation polls have found that Americans now get an average of only about 7 hours.[5] This significant decrease roughly parallels the increase in obesity over the last 50 years. In addition to certain medical or mental health issues (including pain and depression, which are beyond the scope of this book), here are the factors that impact the inability to get a full night's sleep:

- **IGNORING YOUR BODY'S INTERNAL CLOCK.** Our bodies are programmed to be awake during daylight hours and to sleep when the sun goes down—referred to as our circadian rhythm. With the advent of electricity, we now have the ability to override our biological instincts in an effort to get more done.[6]

- **WORK AND COMMUTING.** Many people now choose (or can only afford) to live far from their workplace and may travel up to 1 hour or more each way, 5 days a week. Working evening or night shifts may also make it hard to sleep when the rest of the household is up. Extensive research confirms that working at night also plays havoc with your circadian rhythm.[7] Parents, particularly women, often juggle conflicting work and family responsibilities, cutting into sleep time.

- **AMBIENT NOISE.** Living in an urban environment, or even in a suburban or rural area, perhaps near a firehouse or a stop sign, or close to night owls who blast heavy metal music from their stereo, can definitely interfere with sleep.

- **LIGHT.** Whether it comes from the sun, a light in the hall outside your bedroom, bright streetlights, or car headlights, light is an enemy of sound sleep.[8]

- **ELECTRONIC DEVICES.** Watching television or using a cellphone, computer, or tablet in bed is one of the prime offenders when it comes to diminished or compromised sleep, as we'll discuss in depth in the next chapter. The "blue light" these devices emit is particularly problematic.

- **STRESS.** Ironically, the very devices that were supposed to free up time have actually robbed us of leisure time. Many people are chronically stressed because they feel incapable of handling all their responsibilities in their limited free time. Financial, health, and family concerns are also a source of stress.[9–12]

- **PHYSICAL INACTIVITY.** Sitting around all day can interfere with the body's natural instinct to refuel at night. As we've moved from an industrial society to a data-driven one, most people sit down to do their jobs.[13]

No wonder we're a sleep-deprived society, as robust sales of sleep aids and prescription sleep drugs attest.

ONE-THIRD OF YOUR LIFE

Getting enough sleep is essential, but to awaken refreshed and ready to tackle the new day, we also require quality sleep. If you're getting at least 7 hours of shut-eye a night but wake up frequently or simply don't feel refreshed in the morning, something is interfering with your sleep, whether or not you're aware of it at the time. Some of the same factors that make it hard to fall asleep or stay asleep may also be making your sleep less restorative.

Skimping on sleep causes numerous problems, starting with its short-term impact on your alertness and energy level. It also weakens your body's defenses against infection and increases anxiety, as well as inflammation, the risk of high blood pressure, heart disease, and other chronic illnesses.[14, 15]

When you're exhausted, your immune system is compromised, making you more vulnerable to any germs or viruses that come along.[16] And if you do get sick, it knocks you for a loop in terms of physical activity and even eating properly for a period of time. To compound things, inactivity makes you less likely to rebound from a cold or other virus-borne illness. Lack of sleep can also be a safety issue. According to the Centers for Disease Control and Prevention, one in 24 adults reports having recently fallen asleep at the wheel of a car, and 29 percent of American workers report getting less than 6 hours of sleep a night on average.

It's important to distinguish among the various reasons for being sleep deprived.

If you've gotten in the habit of staying up to stream movies on Netflix or to Skype with friends in different time zones, you've made a voluntary choice to use time that once would have been spent in the sack. If you feel you don't have the time to "waste" in bed because of having to juggle multiple responsibilities, you're still choosing to deal with your to-do list rather than your own well-being. Both of these patterns qualify as voluntary or situational. Hopefully, as you learn how incredibly valuable sleep is, you'll find ways to make other choices. Chances are that you'll find your increased energy will allow you to accomplish more in less time.

On the other hand, insomnia, defined as difficulty falling asleep, waking frequently or too early, falling asleep during the day, or generally experiencing non-restorative sleep, is something else. Even though you're tired and get in bed, sleep eludes you. According to the National Center on Sleep Disorders Research at the National Institutes of Health, 30 to 40 percent of adults experience insomnia from time to time, and 10 to 15 percent of them suffer from chronic insomnia. Moreover, 4 percent of adults rely on a prescription sleep aid, and older people are most apt to do so. If you're dealing with chronic insomnia, some of the suggestions in this chapter will be helpful, but I also advise you to consult a physician.

SLEEP AND WEIGHT

Insufficient sleep leads to weight gain in at least three ways.[17]

1. You don't burn fat for energy as well.

2. Your appetite is increased.

3. You have less energy to be physically active.

Let's look at these one by one.

The hormone insulin is associated with diabetes, but reduced sleep duration increases insulin resistance.[18–21] Remember, the more of this fat-storage hormone you produce, the less glucose you burn for energy and the more body fat you pack on. In the past four decades or so, those of us who live in industrialized societies have gotten less sleep than our parents and grandparents used to get. In that time, there's been a parallel and dramatic increase in the incidence of obesity, among children as well as adults. A growing body of research studies links lack of sleep with insulin resistance and increased risk for obesity.[22, 23] Impaired glucose tolerance can occur even with short-term sleep deprivation.[24]

On the other hand, getting enough sleep is associated with a lower body weight and lower level of body fat. One study that looked at men and women over a 6-year period found that those who went from sleeping less than 6 hours a day to sleeping 7 to 8 hours gained fewer fat pounds than other participants.[25] Another large study that followed subjects over a 5- to 10-year period found a consistent association between the amount of sleep deprivation and obesity. Those who slept less than 7 hours were more likely to be obese.[26] Young adults who had their body mass index (BMI) tested four times over a 13-year period found that the more sleep they got, the lower their ratio of fat to lean body mass.[27]

Still another study that looked at pairs of identical and fraternal twins found that the twin who slept between 7 and almost 9 hours a night had a consistently lower BMI than the twin who regularly slept less.[28] In the case of identical twins, this meant that despite having the same genetic makeup, the amount of sleep each twin got was reflected in the amount of body fat. In each case, the one who got more sleep was slimmer.

There's also very strong association between sleep disturbance and major depression, which is often linked to being overweight.[29-31]

MORE HORMONES AT WORK

So, how does simply getting another hour or so of sleep a night enable you to lose weight? Along with insulin, two other hormones come into play, both of which transmit messages to your brain regarding hunger and satiety.

- Ghrelin, produced in your gastrointestinal tract, is an appetite stimulant. The more ghrelin in your system, the more food you want.

- Leptin, produced in your fat cells, signals your brain when you're full. But when levels of leptin are low, it sends out starvation signals.

As long as everything is working well, levels of these two hormones balance each other so that you neither undereat nor overeat.

However, when you skimp on sleep, leptin levels plummet, meaning you don't feel satisfied, even right after a meal. Simultaneously, lack of sleep causes your ghrelin levels to soar, stimulating your appetite regardless of when you last ate. Obviously, this combination can lead to overeating and excess pounds.[32] That is the last thing you want when your goal is to lose those 5 pounds—fast!

Aside from the hormonal and chemical reactions you experience when you're not getting enough rest, simply being tired impacts other aspects of your life, which can sabotage your weight-loss efforts. You're probably not going to be as physically active when you're exhausted, nor make the smartest eating decisions. And because of the roles of leptin and ghrelin, you're going to have a different palate, different cravings, and less control over knowing when you're full.

Several studies drive home this point dramatically. In one, conducted at the University of Chicago, a dozen healthy young men had their leptin and ghrelin levels measured before being allowed to sleep up to 10 hours for 2 nights. About 6 weeks later, they were allowed only 4 hours of sleep for 2 nights, after which their ghrelin levels were 28 percent higher.[33] Now it gets really interesting. After the short-sleep nights, cravings for fattening, high-carbohydrate, high-calorie foods, such as sweets and salty and starchy foods, increased by 45 percent. Appetite for fruits and vegetables also increased, but not as much nor as consistently. Nor was there any change in the appetite for protein after the short sleep periods. So not only were the sleep-deprived subjects eating more food, but they also craved the very foods likely to pack on pounds.

A much larger study found an almost 15 percent increase in ghrelin levels and a more than 15 percent decrease in leptin levels in people who regularly slept for 5 hours compared with those who slept for 8 hours.[34] The study results also correlated hormone level changes and amount of sleep to weight gain. People displayed an almost 4 percent increase in BMI when their average nightly sleep decreased from 8 to 5 hours.

STILL MORE IMPORTANT HORMONES: MELATONIN AND SEROTONIN

Your pineal gland produces melatonin, the hormone that regulates your body's natural clock (circadian rhythm), which controls the sleep/awake cycle. Melatonin is a neurotransmitter, meaning that it sends messages between nerve cells. You've probably heard of melatonin as a supplement you can take to avoid jet lag when traveling across multiple time zones. Two of the factors that determine how much melatonin your body makes are your body clock and your exposure to light. You can control the latter to a certain extent, but not the former. Melatonin levels normally begin to rise in the evening and stay high for most of the night. Then they go down in the early morning. In winter, shorter days impact how much and when melatonin is produced. This is one reason why it's important to spend at least 20 minutes outdoors every day. And the more sunshine you get and the earlier in the day you do so, the more likely you are to be slim, according to a new study.[35]

Another neurotransmitter, serotonin is often referred to as the feel-good hormone. Increased levels make you feel relaxed, which helps you fall asleep, among other effects. But serotonin, along with other hormones, can be disrupted by stress and erratic sleep habits. Eating a meal that includes foods high in the amino acid tryptophan, such as turkey and other meats, cheese and other dairy products, and nuts and seeds, in combination with carbohydrate-rich foods, can help raise serotonin levels.

THE STRESS HORMONE

Cortisol is yet another hormone impacted by sleep deprivation. Produced by your adrenal gland, cortisol is known as the stress hormone. Under normal conditions, cortisol levels begin to decrease quickly as evening approaches and reach their lowest levels at the time you usually go to bed. However, when sleep is restricted, this natural process is interrupted.[36, 37] In one study in which subjects had their sleep reduced for almost a week, the rate at which their cortisol levels decreased was about six times slower than it was in subjects who were fully rested.[38]

Chronic sleep loss leading to higher-than-normal evening cortisol levels doesn't just make you more subject to stress; it also likely contributes to the development of insulin resistance, which, as we've already discussed, puts you at risk for obesity. If you're feeling more stressed at night from elevated cortisol levels, you'll likely find it hard to fall asleep. If you have trouble sleeping night after night, your cortisol levels will rise still more, compounding the storage of body fat.

Sleep and Your Diet

Getting enough sleep is intimately linked to adopting a healthy diet, another reminder of the synergy of My 5. The less you sleep, the more likely you are to eat fats and refined carbohydrates, and the less likely to consume vegetables and fruits. You're also more likely to have irregular meal patterns than people who sleep more. People who are starved for sleep are more apt to skip breakfast than those who get a minimum of 7 hours of shut-eye.[39] Eating mostly snacks and/or eating late at night also correlates with short sleep sessions.[40] Clearly, such habits are a recipe for weight gain.

Follow the food and beverage guidelines below to improve your sleeping habits, which will in turn help you shed 5 pounds in a week, as promised.[41]

- Avoid caffeinated products, alcohol, and nicotine for 4 hours before bedtime.
- Avoid large meals in the evening.
- Don't skip dinner.
- Avoid too many fluids prior to bedtime.
- Avoid highly spiced, heavy, or sugary foods at nighttime.
- Drink a cup of chamomile, linden flower, peppermint, or other herbal tea before bed.
- Consume magnesium-rich foods such as broccoli, nuts, oysters, scallops, squash, and wheat bread as part of your diet.

LIGHT FANTASTIC

Early-morning sunlight is your best prescription for sound sleep that night. The ancients were on to something with morning salutations honoring the god of light! Here's another powerful motivator to get out early for a walk. A new study found that people who got 20 to 30 minutes of sunlight before noon had a significantly lower BMI than those who got their exposure later in the day.[42] Results were independent of the level of physical activity, intake of calories, bedtime hour, or length of sleep. The study authors calculated that the timing of light accounted for 20 percent of the resulting BMI.

Incandescent lighting is an acceptable substitute for the sun's rays in bad weather or during the winter. But like so many things in life, timing is everything. Bright light at the end of the day interferes with sleep. It's also associated with a number of health issues.[43] Remember, your internal clock is winding down by dusk. One study found that gradually shifting the time at which subjects were exposed to light, and thus upsetting their circadian rhythm, caused elevated blood sugar levels and reduced levels of leptin.[44] Both effects are likely to result in weight gain.

Nor is it just bright light at the end of the day that scrambles our internal clock. Sitting beside a lighted table lamp before bed can make it more difficult to nod off.[45] Even a nightlight can interfere with sleep. "Blue light" emitted by most electronic devices is the most powerful suppressor of melatonin. Some energy-efficient lightbulbs have similar effects. After exposure to more than 6 hours of blue light, the circadian rhythms of subjects in one study had shifted forward 3 hours.[46, 47] (We'll go into greater detail about this kind of light in the next chapter.) In the meantime, note that in 2012 the American Medical Association issued a policy saying that "exposure to excessive light at night, including extended use of various electronic media, can disrupt sleep or exacerbate sleep disorders."

To keep your internal clock in sync, modify or develop some new nighttime habits:

Excess Weight and Sleep Apnea

Sleep apnea is a serious condition in which a person stops breathing for several seconds, often gasping for breath and disrupting sleep. It's more common in people who are overweight. Sleep apnea can aggravate ongoing sleep deficits and impair sleep quality. It can also create a vicious cycle in which the sleep deprivation causes weight gain, which in turn increases the severity of the apnea and further impacts the quality of sleep, contributing to more weight gain. Also, the heavier you are, the more likely you are to snore, which can awaken you, similarly impacting sleep quality and duration.

- If you use a nightlight, get one with a red light, which is least likely to suppress melatonin production.

- Instead of turning on a light if you need to visit the bathroom, keep a flashlight on your bedside table.

- Turn off the computer, TV, cellphone, and other such devices at least 1 hour before bedtime.

- Don't nod off in front of the television in the evening. It's a sure-fire way to find you can't fall back asleep when you get in bed.

SLEEP AND YOUR BRAIN

Being deprived of sleep, even for just a single night, has a dramatic influence on your brain. In one fascinating study, subjects arrived at a sleep lab well rested. They were presented with images of 80 foods, which they rated on a scale of 1 to 4 in terms of desirability. Brain scans were also done. After a night of sleep deprivation, the subjects were shown the same images and told they could have any food that they rated highly. This time sweet or starchy carbohydrate foods got a bigger response from the amygdala, the part of the brain that controls the impulse to eat. Meanwhile, the frontal cortex, which weighs consequences and makes rational decisions, showed less activity on the brain scans.[48] Matthew P. Walker, one of the study's authors and a professor of psychology and neuroscience at the University of California, Berkeley, referred to this as a "double hit." Being sleep deprived makes you respond more strongly to junk food at the same time your impulse control is weakened.

Sleep deprivation can result in almost immediate weight gain. A recent study at the University of Colorado showed that losing just a few hours of sleep for 5 nights (a typical workweek) in a row caused people to gain an astounding 2 pounds on average.[49] The researchers concluded that although the subjects burned more calories simply by being awake longer, they consumed far more calories than what was needed to offset that extra expenditure of energy. Just

Besieged by Your Bladder

The need to urinate frequently can play havoc with your sleep, whether it's caused by prostate problems, pregnancy, or menopause. In addition to not drinking fluids close to bedtime, talk to your doctor to rule out a serious problem. He or she may suggest medication that could help moderate the urge and/or address the underlying cause. And if your mate is the one getting up every few hours, it is most likely impacting the quality of your sleep too.

getting less sleep doesn't *cause* weight gain. But changes in our brains when we're sleep deprived somehow ignore the normal signals of how much energy (calories) we actually need.

According to Kenneth P. Wright Jr., MD, the director of the University of Colorado–Boulder's Sleep and Chronobiology Laboratory and an author of the study, one factor that may play a role in the connection between lack of sleep and excessive hunger is adenosine. As this by-product of metabolism accumulates in our brain, it promotes sleepiness. While we sleep, adenosine is cleared from the brain. (One of the ways that caffeine keeps us awake is that it blocks adenosine.) When we don't get enough sleep, the adenosine builds up and may interfere with neural communication in the brain. Just as your dishwasher removes gunk from pots and pans, sleep cleans up the toxins in the brain. Our brain, to say nothing about the rest of us, needs to recharge itself after about 16 hours of being "on call."

THE GOOD NEWS

Where does all this research leave you as you try to shed those pesky last 5 pounds—or kick-start a weight-loss program? By establishing good sleeping patterns, meaning at least 7 and preferably 8 hours of sleep a night, you'll:

- Have more control of your appetite because your levels of the hormones ghrelin and leptin are more balanced

- Improve your ability to burn calories more efficiently

- Help nip in the bud insulin resistance, which can lead to weight gain

- Have more energy to be physically active

Beyond this first week on the My 5 Plan, there's more good news. Establishing the habit of regularly getting enough sleep also:

- Helps minimize the amount of weight you'll gain as you age[50]

- Helps reduce your risk factor for disease

- Enhances the likelihood you'll live longer

SET THE SCENE FOR SLEEP

How do you go about improving your sleep habits? Like everything else, practice makes perfect. Get in the habit of going to bed and arising at the same time every day. Sleeping more than 2 to 3 extra hours a night on weekends disrupts your circadian clock. Also don't engage in vigorous physical activity, such as running or spinning, for at least 90 minutes before bedtime. Create a quiet, relaxing environment in your bedroom by removing any distractions and controlling light and noise. Here's how to make your bedroom a refuge:

- Use your bed only for sleeping and sex.

- Remove the TV, computers, and other electronic gadgetry, as well as anything else that induces stress, such as household bills or work. Just having a stress trigger nearby can induce anxiety.

- If you use a digital alarm clock, keep it at least 3 feet away from you and angle it so you can't see the display.

- Use a white noise device if ambient noise is a problem.

- Hang light-blocking curtains or shades.

Turn Down the Heat

Leaving the heat too high at night or piling too many blankets on the bed can make you perspire, disrupting sleep. You want to feel snug when you get in bed and then to cool down during the night, which helps you burn fat while you sleep. But an extremely cold room could also make it difficult to sleep. To get it right:

1. Turn down the thermostat to 70°F or less, perhaps 5 degrees south of its daytime setting.

2. Place two lightweight blankets or quilts, rather than one heavy one, on the bed. You can easily remove one during the night if you get overheated.

3. Bedding made of breathable materials such as cotton, wool, or down allows your body heat to disperse, unlike polyester and other synthetics, which hold it In and can make you perspire and feel clammy.

4. Unless you sleep in the nude, wear nightclothes made of fabrics that breathe to avoid overheating. Tight clothing can also raise your body temperature.

5. If you sleep on a foam mattress, cover it with a cotton pad to wick away perspiration.

BEGIN TO WIND DOWN
BEFORE BEDTIME

The process of falling asleep quickly begins at least an hour before you actually climb into bed. Establish a regular pre-bedtime routine to help speed sleep once you tuck in for the night:

- Take a warm bath or gentle shower, perhaps using soothing lavender-scented bath products.

- Do some easy stretching or gentle yoga or Pilates, which have been shown to cut the amount of time it takes to fall asleep and to help you awake refreshed.[51–56]

- Meditate or practice self-relaxation exercises.

- Play soothing music, which reduces stress and therefore cortisol levels. Music has been shown to increase the amount of REM sleep and shorten stage 2 sleep.[57]

- Read a (regular) book or an e-reader that isn't backlit or listen to a book on tape. The type of light in some tablets, including the iPad, stimulates your brain.

DEVICES TO HELP YOU DOZE

A number of products can improve the quality of your sleep, ranging from low-tech earplugs to block out your partner's snores to the latest digital sleep monitors.

- *Earplugs* can control exposure to noise and therefore improve the length and quality of sleep.[58, 59] They can reduce wakefulness and elevate melatonin levels, although effectiveness varies depending on the type of earplug.[60-63] Noise also diminishes REM sleep; earplugs can increase deep, restorative sleep.

- *Sleep masks* reduce exposure to light, similarly improving sleep length and quality by increasing REM time and raising melatonin levels.[64, 65]

- *Sound-masking devices* use soothing, steady sounds such as of ocean waves (white noise) to block out ambient noise and promote longer periods of deep sleep. Studies have shown that the use of white noise devices improved the quality of sleep in hospital patients by more than 37 percent and in healthy adults by more than 67 percent, in both cases compared with a control group that didn't use such devices.[66-68]

- *Sleep monitors* record both the length and the quality of your sleep by detecting movements of your wrist. (Others come with a headband.

What is REM Sleep?

Rapid eye movement (REM) sleep accounts for about one-quarter of normal sleep and is associated with dreaming. Periods of REM sleep tend to last longer as morning approaches. The remaining three-quarters of our sleep is non-rapid eye movement (NREM) sleep, which consists of four stages, ranging from stage 1 (light sleep) to stage 4 (deep sleep).

Some trackers, including Aura and Beddit, are placed under your bottom sheet.) Many activity monitors, such as the Fitbit Flex, are also sleep monitors. They record how long it takes you to fall asleep, how long you are actually asleep, and how often you wake up (some of which you may not remember in the morning), as well as your pulse rate. Your blood oxygen levels could signal whether you have sleep apnea. More sophisticated models also measure your REM sleep periods.[69] The monitor wirelessly sends data to your computer. Understanding your sleep patterns is the first step to making changes to improve sleep quality. You can buy a basic activity/sleep monitor for about $100.

- *A continuous positive airway pressure (CPAP) device* allows people who suffer from sleep apnea to breathe unobstructed and maintain healthy blood oxygen levels. A face mask or nasal piece creates a vacuum around the nose, while a plastic hose delivers a steady stream of air. While it can seem awkward at first, once you adapt to a CPAP device, it can relieve such symptoms as waking up struggling for breath, snoring, and low respiratory rates. If you suffer from sleep apnea, your doctor can prescribe a CPAP device, the cost of which is typically covered by health insurance.

MAKE YOUR BEDROOM A DRUG-FREE ZONE

According to a 2013 Centers for Disease Control and Prevention report, about 4 percent of Americans had taken a prescription sleep aid in the previous month, and women are significantly more likely to use them than men. Americans now spend close to $5 billion a year on sleep medications such as Ambien, Lunesta, Sonata, Halcion, and Restoril.[70, 71] (Each pill costs up to $4!) So, how effective are these pricey pills? When tested against a placebo, Ambien, Lunesta, and Sonata, which are relatively new products, enabled users to get to sleep 13 minutes faster.[72]

Not very impressive, is it? Even less impressive is that the pill takers got only about 11 more minutes of sleep than did those taking a placebo. Halcion and Restoril, which are older medications, did slightly better: Those who took the drugs dozed off 10 minutes faster than those on a placebo and slept 32 minutes longer. Interestingly, the subjects *thought* that they had slept longer than they actually did: 32 extra minutes instead of 11 on the newer drugs, and 52 extra minutes on the older drugs.

Why the discrepancy? One of the side effects of taking sleeping pills is anterograde amnesia.[73] This condition interferes with the ability to form memories. In other words, the test subjects may have simply forgotten that they had been unable to sleep. In addition to morning drowsiness, sleeping

The Right Mattress

Research indicates that only 7 percent of sleep problems are the result of an uncomfortable mattress.[74, 75] However, if you're tired and achy in the morning or your mattress is more than 7 years old, you may need to replace it. Likewise, if you can see the imprint of your body or you're rolling into the center, it's time. But will spending more for a mattress give you a proportionally better night's sleep? You can buy a Serta innerspring queen-size mattress for about $1,000, while a Duxiana of the same size (with box spring) goes for about $7,000. However, according to *Consumer Reports*, which puts mattresses through extensive tests before rating them, price has little to do with quality.

Most people are comfortable on a medium-firm mattress, which supports the spine and allows it to maintain its natural curve. Research bears this out. One study showed that a medium-firm mattress improved sleep quality by 55 percent.[76] Too firm a mattress won't support all parts of your body evenly. A mattress that's so soft you sink into it could restrict movement, meaning you could wake up stiff and achy. You also want a firm enough edge so you won't roll out of bed at night. As long as you can sit securely on the bed to put on your socks and shoes, you're fine.

Would you buy a new car without test-driving it? Of course not. So don't even consider buying a new mattress without giving it a "spin." Spend at least 15 minutes lying on your side as well as on your back before making a decision. A recent *Consumer Reports* subscriber survey of in-store testers found that about 75 percent of those who "test-drove" the mattress at a store before making their purchase said the mattress helped improve their sleep.

Pillow Talk

The right pillow can make all the difference between waking refreshed and ready to take on the world or starting the day with an achy neck, arm, or shoulder. There's no one perfect pillow for everyone. Your side-sleeping mate may love a soft pillow, while you, a committed back-sleeper, may prefer a firm one. One thing's for sure. If your pillow is more than 2 years old, it's worn out its usefulness. If you're still clinging to an old pillow, it's probably full of dust mites, your own skin cells, and other yucky things. Think about the following when buying a new pillow:

- **MATERIAL.** Choose down, a down-feather mix, or polyester memory foam.

- **QUALITY.** Look for even distribution of the filling, straight seams, and a zipper.

- **FIRMNESS.** The more pressure you need to apply to a pillow, the firmer it is. The faster it returns to its original height, the more resilient it is.

- **PRICE.** The cost of a memory-foam pillow doesn't seem to affect quality, but when it comes to down pillows, price does appear to correlate with comfort, according to *Consumer Reports*.

- **ODOR.** Both memory foam and down products may need to be aired out for several days before using.

Finally, be sure to purchase a zippered cover to extend the life of your pillow.

pills have been linked to some serious although rare side effects, including sleepwalking, raiding the fridge while asleep, and even sleep driving!

The most common side effect of such drugs is morning drowsiness. But a long list of others includes burning or tingling sensations in your extremities, constipation, diarrhea, loss of balance, dizziness, dry mouth, gas, headache, heartburn, shakiness, vivid dreams, and weakness. Read the labels and you'll see that depression is another side effect. People who rely on sleeping pills often end up also taking an antidepressant. They may also be prescribed a mood stabilizer. So now, to get a few more minutes of sleep and to fall asleep a bit faster, they're taking three prescription medications. When you consider how ineffective and dangerous sleeping pills can be, it's hard to understand why anyone without a serious medical condition would put his or her health at risk when there are more natural approaches like those discussed in these pages.

WHO ARE YOU SLEEPING WITH?

Your sleepmate, whether human, canine, feline, or a combination thereof, may play an unintended role in how well you're sleeping. Here are the two most common problems and some ways to address them:

- **LOVE YOUR MATE, HATE HIS/HER SNORING.** If you can't convince your partner to sleep on his/her side, which reduces the likelihood of snoring, check out the single-use strips worn on the bridge of the nose that open the nasal passages and can help reduce the racket. An old trick is to put a tennis ball in a T-shirt with a pocket, and then have the sleeper wear it backward to keep from rolling over. Mouth guards that reposition the jaw are another possibility. If all else fails, simply take yourself to the guest room on those nights when it becomes too much. Discuss this ahead of time to avoid hurt feelings. According to Jordan Josephson, MD, a nasal and endoscopic sinus surgeon at Lenox Hill Hospital in New York City, snoring and sleep apnea are the number-one medical cause of relationship breakups and divorce.[77] Chronic snoring can indicate a serious health issue and should be brought to the attention of your doctor.

- **FED UP WITH FURRY FRIENDS?** According to a recent survey by the American Pet Products Association, 62 percent of small dogs, 32 percent of large dogs, and 62 percent of cats sleep with their owners. While pets provide warmth and affection, they can hog the bed and snore, just like our human bedmates. They can also introduce allergens that interfere with sleep. It may be time to move them to another room or at least to their own beds on the floor.

DAYTIME STRATEGIES FOR NIGHTTIME BLISS

A number of small decisions you make throughout the day can pay big dividends come nightfall. These habits will help:

- **OPEN THE CURTAINS OR PULL UP THE SHADES AS SOON AS YOU GET UP.** Every little bit of morning light helps. Remember, the more natural light you get, the more your internal clock stays in sync, which is essential to regulating your core body temperature and melatonin levels.[78]

- **TAKE BREAKS OUTDOORS WHENEVER POSSIBLE.** Ideally, you should get at least 30 minutes of morning light each day, which can help address insomnia.[79–82]

- **MOVE YOUR DESK CLOSE TO A WINDOW.** Take advantage of natural light if possible.

- **USE A LIGHT THERAPY BOX.** If you live in a northern climate and experience seasonal affective disorder (SAD), a light therapy box will help to sync your internal clock.

- **BE ACTIVE.** Taking 10,000 steps a day helps people with insomnia sleep longer and wake up more refreshed than those who don't walk as much.[83]

- **ENGAGE WITH OTHER PEOPLE REGULARLY.** Social isolation can interfere with healthy sleep habits and promote stress, but social interaction can provide a sense of belonging and emotional support, which can encourage good sleep habits.[84] Feeling purposeful—that your life has meaning—is also associated with sleep duration and amount of REM sleep.[85]

- **COUNT YOUR BLESSINGS.** In one study, people who did so weekly for 10 weeks displayed fewer physical complaints, spent more time exercising and sleeping, and experienced better-quality sleep than those who didn't count their blessings.[86, 87]

- **TAKE A CATNAP.** But limit it to 30 minutes and do it early in the afternoon.

GETTING BACK TO SLEEP

If you find yourself unable to fall back asleep after waking during the night, try these tactics:

- Focus on your body instead of your mind. The more you stress about being unable to sleep, the more the stress will keep you awake. Cue yourself to relax, perhaps progressively starting with your toes and slowly moving up to your head. Enjoy the warmth of your covers, the silkiness of the sheets, and the peacefulness of the darkened room. By focusing on relaxation instead of sleep, you may take the pressure off yourself to fall asleep. Relaxation may then breed sleep.

- Visualize yourself in a peaceful place (or counting sheep jumping over a fence, if you prefer) or practice deep breathing or meditation.

- Put off brainstorming. Keep a pencil and pad by the bed so that if you come up with a great idea in the middle of the night, you can jot it down and not have to worry that you'll forget it by morning. Likewise, if you're worrying about something, acknowledge it on the pad and rest assured that you'll deal with it the next day.

- If you don't doze off within 20 minutes, leave the bedroom and do something relaxing in dim light in another room. Return to bed only when you're nodding off.

Let me reiterate the importance of unplugging as the day comes to a close. Turn off your phone and other technology at night. Not only is it important to not have these screens emitting light, but there is also something symbolic about it. For me, shutting down my phone or disabling the antenna so it doesn't receive any calls, e-mails, or texts marks the end of my day. And just in case I have to remind you, all this focus on sleep, beds, bedmates, and the like is to help you slim down fast!

In the next chapter, we'll explore the fifth and last part of the My 5 Plan, which is all about unplugging from our wonderful but intrusive electronic world.

Five Key Points in Chapter 4

1. Getting less than 7 hours of continuous sleep a night (or experiencing poor-quality sleep) can significantly hamper weight-loss efforts for a number of reasons. You're inclined to eat more, especially refined carbohydrates, when sleep deprived. There's a clear association between sleep deprivation and a higher BMI.

2. Several hormones can create a perfect storm for weight gain. When you're not well rested, your insulin response may be suppressed, increasing the likelihood of storing fat rather than burning it. Levels of ghrelin, an appetite stimulant, also rise, while levels of leptin, which signals satiety, decrease. Levels of the stress hormone cortisol also rise.

3. Melatonin is another key hormone to good sleep. Your body produces melatonin during the day. Low melatonin levels at bedtime make it difficult to fall asleep.

4. Modern life has interrupted our natural body clock, or circadian rhythms. Spending too much time in front of electronic devices that emit blue light also messes with your body's internal clock.

5. Establishing regular bedtime habits, getting enough exercise, exposing yourself to sunlight or other light, and eating a diet low in refined carbohydrates are all integral to falling asleep and staying asleep. All are part of the My 5 Plan.

CHAPTER

PULL THE CORD

Isn't living in the digital age wonderful? We have instant access to all kinds of information, a multitude of ways to connect with far-flung friends and family, and a vast shopping mall we can visit day or night without leaving the house. You can even get a college degree online! But have you ever wondered what all the lights on our electronic devices, the glare from the TV or computer screen, and the ring, ring, ring of our cellphones are doing to your nerves and your body? And could these devices that connect you to this vast virtual world also be connected to your weight issues? Hold that thought.

How many hours a day do you spend at your computer, whether checking e-mail, shopping, checking out YouTube, or seeing what your friends are up to on Facebook? How about time spent talking, texting, tweeting, shooting videos, and sending photos on your cellphone? And what about watching your favorite shows on TV or online? Are you constantly checking out cable news? Do you play video games? Tally your hours of screen time and I suspect you'll be surprised. And we're not even talking about using your computer at work.

Consider these shocking statistics:[1]

- The average American spends more than 4 hours a day watching television, and older viewers watch even more.

- Sixty-six percent of Americans regularly watch television while eating dinner.

- Adults now spend about 60 hours a week consuming all forms of electronic media, some of it duplicative—texting while watching TV, for example. That's more time than we spend sleeping!

- Only 12 percent of mobile phone use is spent talking and texting.

One of the ways we pay for our comfortable lifestyle is with the thickness of our collective waistline. A multicountry study involving almost 154,000 adults found that the higher the rate of ownership of computers and TVs in each country, the lower its citizens' level of physical activity, the more hours spent sitting, the greater the number of calories consumed, and the higher the average BMI.[2]

SET YOURSELF FREE

This brings us to the final component of My 5: unplugging from all the electronic devices we're so (literally) attached to. Don't panic. I'm not talking about altogether, just for at least 1 consecutive hour a day. Yes, these devices provide an array of great services, but the flip side is that they run the risk of dominating our lives. Once you do detach yourself for 60 minutes from the clutter of input that rules most of your waking hours, you'll be amazed at how your mind quiets, your stress recedes, and you find time to pursue activities you'd pushed aside. It's also surprisingly easy to do.

We've discussed how driving, rather than walking or taking public transportation, has made us a plumper, more sedentary population. Now let's look at the connection between our electronic media habits and our weight. The largest risk of spending too much time in the virtual world is that it inherently fosters inactivity and cuts into time that could be better spent on more

5 Five Ways Watching TV Makes You Fat

1. It displaces time spent being physically active.

2. It provides more opportunities for unhealthy snacking.

3. It distracts you, leading to mindless eating.

4. It can cut into sleep time, which can lead to weight gain.[3]

5. Blue light emissions (see page 108) suppress melatonin production, which interferes with sleep.

active pursuits. That's a double whammy weight-wise. As you now know, an hour at the gym isn't going to compensate for hours of sitting on your bum staring at the screen. Toss into the mix the poor eating habits often associated with watching TV, and we have a triple whammy. And of course, as we just discussed in Chapter 4, using electronic devices can also cut into your sleep time, which compounds the impact on your weight. It's all connected!

THE BIG SCREEN

Although small-screen devices are grabbing an increasingly large slice of the screen-time pie, television viewing still has an enormous impact on our collective weight. Watching TV is almost always a seated "activity." Thanks to the invention of the remote (and now voice recognition), you need barely move for hours, other than taking bathroom breaks or raiding the fridge. Television usage is the most heavily researched form of electronic media simply because it's been around the longest, but many of the findings apply to the other devices as well. Viewing habits are changing: More people, particularly younger folks, are now watching movies and television shows on their computers, tablets, and smartphones. So the number of TV hours may continue to decline, but it's unlikely that total screen time will diminish. If anything, recent trends indicate that it's likely to increase.

WHAT YOU VIEW
AND WHAT YOU CHEW

There's mounting evidence that watching television (and using other devices) has significantly changed what, when, and how we eat. The mere fact that we're eating while focusing on something else promotes "mindless eating," making us more likely to overeat and to make poor food choices both while we're watching TV and afterward.[4–13] Snacking while watching television is the norm for many people. Just think about the brouhaha about what to serve at Super Bowl get-togethers. Place any snack food in close proximity to the TV and it's likely to get eaten whether or not viewers are actually hungry.[14] And then there's the two-thirds of the population who dine most nights in front of the TV.

Mindless eating also impairs your ability to accurately estimate the amount of food you've eaten.[15] It makes people unintentionally consume more calories, fat, and sugary, starchy foods than they would otherwise, greatly increasing their chances of becoming overweight. On the other hand, mindful eating is key to eating moderately. A review of two dozen earlier studies revealed that people watching TV consume more than those who don't eat in front of the screen.[16]

Finally, images of junk food ads parade across the screen at every station break. The practice of food product placements in TV shows sends subtle but consistent messages. Sitting down, eating mindlessly in front of a screen, and receiving frequent reminders to eat more red licorice, sugar-encrusted cereals, peanut butter cups, burgers, batter-fried fish, and other foods high in calories and low in vitamins and minerals are a dangerous combination.

Children and teens are particularly vulnerable to food advertising. Much of the research linking television viewing with consuming more calories or making poor food and beverage choices has focused on children and adolescents. It strongly suggests that ads for junk food, overall TV viewing, and the increase in childhood and adolescent obesity are intimately linked. (See "Plugged-In Kids" on page 107.) But studies on adults confirm similar results: The more time logged in front of the TV, the more likely adults are to gain weight or become overweight or obese.[17] In fact, there's a direct association between the number of hours logged in front of the TV and amount of body weight, again, in part because watching TV replaces physical activities.[18]

MORE HOURS, MORE POUNDS

As we've discussed, the more time you spend watching TV or using a computer, the more likely you are to be heavy. One small study gave some adults the opportunity to use a lockout device that cut television viewing by half and compared their weight-loss efforts with those of a control group with no limits on TV watching. People who used the device watched less television and burned more daily calories than the control group.[19] A study of more than 42,600 Canadian adults found that those who spent 21 or more hours a week watching TV were almost twice as likely to be obese as those who watched 5 or fewer hours a week.[20]

Sadly, women seem to get the short end of the stick here. Some research suggests that heavy TV viewing and a sedentary lifestyle are more consistently associated with being overweight for women than for men.[21] When more than 50,000 women, none of whom were initially obese, were tracked over a 6-year period, for every 2 additional hours a week spent in front of the TV, their risk for obesity increased by 23 percent.[22]

Watching TV But Not *the* TV

A 2014 survey of the media consumption and technology habits of more than 2,000 people reveals that younger millennials (people in their teens and early twenties) are more apt to watch movies and television shows on their computers, smartphones, and tablets than on a television.[23] According to consulting firm Deloitte, which commissioned the survey, Generation X, baby boomers, and mature viewers continue to watch most movies and TV shows the conventional way. Older millennials (ages 25 to 30) also still use the television more than 50 percent of the time. But the trend is clear. Ninety percent of viewers claim they watch some video content online, in large part on tablets, but also on computers and smartphones.[24]

Reducing sedentary habits, including watching TV, has the potential to increase life expectancy, according to an analysis of the respected National Health and Nutrition Examination Survey.[25] Cutting the time spent sitting to less than 3 hours a day is estimated to increase average life span by 2 years. Cutting TV time to less than 2 hours a day can add another 1.38 years. Reducing all sitting time, as well as breaking up sedentary periods, will also likely reduce your likelihood of weight gain and associated health risks.[26]

THE COMPUTER AGE

Among younger people at least, the computer is replacing the TV as the screen venue of choice. But whether you're watching movies and TV shows or writing a thesis, it doesn't change the implications for your weight. Using either device almost always involves sitting, often for hours at a time. A standing or adjustable desk can help remedy the situation, but sitting isn't the only health threat associated with computer use. When 25,000 Japanese employees who worked at computers filled out questionnaires over a 3-year period for a study, they reported depression, anxiety, irritation with coworkers, and reluctance to go to work, along with problems sleeping and daytime fatigue.[27] The researchers concluded that working at a computer for more than 5 hours a day significantly increased mental health and sleep-related problems.

Several similar surveys of computer professionals at software companies in India found that long-term computer use resulted in vision problems, back pain, and other musculoskeletal pain, as well as weight gain and stress.[28-31] There's also concern that sitting at a computer for long periods could result in deep-vein thrombosis, which is more commonly associated with prolonged airplane flights. That's another powerful incentive to get up and move around several times an hour when using any electronic device.

Whether you use a computer for work, leisure activities, or both, the amount of time you're immobile links directly to the risk for being

A Global Phenomenon

The United States may have the highest obesity rate, but other developed nations are catching up fast. In "Waistlines of the World: The Effect of Information and Communications Technology on Obesity," authors Anusuya Chatterjee and Ross C. DeVol explore the global impact of increased portion sizes, a sedentary lifestyle, and less strenuous work over the past 20 years.[32] They write, "In the past two decades, there has been a worldwide transition toward an 'information/knowledge-based society' that led to changes in work habits and lifestyle. As a side effect, people started consuming more calories than they expended, which resulted in weight gain and obesity." The authors posit that for every 10 percent increase in investment in communications technology, there is a 1 percent increase in obesity, compounded by a further 0.4 percent increase thanks to more time in front of a screen for a total 1.4 percent increase in obesity. That may not sound too bad, but for a country with a population of 300 million, that means 4.2 million newly obese citizens. And if technology continues to develop at the pace it has over the past two decades, those numbers will keep increasing.

overweight. For example, a study of more than 2,600 Australian adults found that those who reported high computer or Internet leisure time use were one and a half times more likely to be overweight and slightly more than two and a half times more likely to be obese than participants who used neither.[33] Even Internet and computer users who also engage in physical activities in their leisure time were far more likely to be overweight or obese than those who didn't use a computer during their nonwork hours. As discussed in Chapter 2, research shows that working out at a gym or engaging in other forms of traditional exercise doesn't compensate for the effects of sitting for extended periods of time.

Some enlightened companies are coming up with ways to help their employees unplug and get away from their desks for breaks, along with making other health-conscious changes in the corporate culture. For example, Huffington Post Media Group now has nap rooms and opportunities for workers to meditate or do yoga or breathing exercises. In a talk at Princeton University, CEO Arianna Huffington spoke of her own breakdown from stress and overwork and how it has changed her philosophy about what constitutes success and the work environment. "Thirty-five percent [of companies] have introduced some form of stress reduction policies," she said. "The cost of burnout is convincing companies to change their practices. We can't just be in a reacting mode, dealing with smartphones and other people's needs. We have to have quiet time to create. Increasing creativity is necessary in a job."[34]

SOCIAL MEDIA AND EMOTIONAL HEALTH

Computer use encompasses everything from researching your genealogy to watching cat videos. But one particular activity, whether pursued on a computer, tablet, or smartphone, has its own implications for emotional health. For all its ability to connect people worldwide, social networking can provoke anxiety and a sense of isolation. Do I have as many friends on Facebook as my sister-in-law does? Why does no one ever retweet my tweets? Why does my cell ping so rarely? Why does my friend's blog have so many more followers than mine? Why are so few "matches" getting back to me on that dating site I joined?

Heavy use of Facebook and other social media sites can play a role in depression, particularly among adolescents, who are more subject to peer pressure and the influence of online media than adults.[35] But adults, too, can

From Pull to Push

Talk about TMI (too much information)! Have you noticed that your incoming e-mails, texts, tweets, and other electronic message seem to be multiplying? You're not imagining things. In the past 3 years, there's been a sea change on the Internet. It used to be that *you* would take the initiative to search for information, known as "pull" usership. Now marketers increasingly take the initiative to push information on you, based on algorithms compiled from data on your user habits. "Push" usership has made it almost impossible to escape the delivery of information you may not want. This phenomenon is yet another reason to unplug for at least an hour a day.

be subject to depression and feelings of inadequacy from social media. A survey by *The Today Show* is a case in point. Among more than 7,000 mothers who use Pinterest, a site on which users can share photos of their projects, 42 percent of them admitted to occasional "Pinterest stress." How come? They felt that their creative efforts weren't as impressive as those of other posters, who appeared to have "perfect" lives. Women are more likely to suffer from stress and depression generated by their social media experiences than men. Although it's hard to establish cause and effect, it's well known that depression and obesity are often associated.

Not all people engaging in social media feel depressed, stressed, or inadequate, of course. Use of social networking sites has also been shown to *reinforce* social bonds for college students,[36] as well as the elderly, who may feel socially isolated. One study of 8,000 men and women aged 50 and above found that Internet and social media users are 30 percent *less likely* to experience depression than nonusers.[37]

MORE MEDIA, MORE OF THE TIME

A new trend is emerging: the simultaneous use of a smartphone, computer or tablet, and the television, also known as media multitasking. In 2013, Accenture, a management consulting company, released the results of its third annual Video-Over-Internet online poll on viewing habits, which surveyed more than 3,500 consumers in six countries, including the United States.[38] Of these, more than three-quarters said they regularly use their laptop computer *while* watching TV, up from 61 percent just a year earlier; and 68 percent use a smartphone. Although not as many people own tablets as smartphones or laptops, the simultaneous use of television and tablets had mushroomed from 11 percent to 44 percent in one year. Simultaneous television and game console use leaped from 9 to 34 percent over a year.

The Deloitte survey on viewing habits I mentioned earlier found that about 86 percent of viewers were multitasking, watching TV while going to another screen to check their e-mail, text, use a social network, or browse the Web. Meanwhile, research shows that increased media multi-tasking is associated with higher rates of depression and social anxiety symptoms.[39] However, it's unclear whether multitasking causes such symptoms or whether depressed or anxious people engage in it to distract themselves from their problems. If television viewing is strongly corre-lated with inactivity and the risk for obesity, what's the impact of this new paradigm of simultaneous use of electronic devices? It might actually decrease rather than increase sitting time, as people often pace around while on a cellphone.

Plugged-In Kids

Consider these disturbing findings from the research focused on the younger generation:

- **TELEVISION.** Study after study shows that the more screen time kids rack up, the heavier they are on average[40-44] and the more likely they are to wind up as fat adults.[45, 46] Increased viewing has also been tied to poor sleep and school performance.[47, 48] Excessive television viewing and video games are also associated with an increase in attention deficit disorders in children,[49] as well as increased calorie intake,[50, 51] obesity, and poor dietary habits.[52-54] Not surprisingly, hav-ing a TV in a youngster's bedroom leads to more viewing hours and a greater likelihood of poor school performance.[55] The good news is that when parents restrict the time kids spend in front of the television and computer and monitor the content, there are multiple positive effects: more sleep, better performance in school, improved behavior, and a more favorable BMI.[56]

- **CELLPHONES.** A study of almost 29,000 Danish kids showed a sig-nificantly higher risk for behavioral problems among young children who used mobile phones and whose mothers also used them during pregnancy.[57]

- **VIDEO GAMES.** Ninety percent of kids play video games. Violent games are associated with aggressive behavior.[58] So-called active video games are designed so that players must move around to con-trol the screen. A small study suggests that replacing sedentary video games with active ones may help overweight kids reduce their BMI.[59]

BLUE LIGHT, SLEEP, AND WEIGHT

In the last chapter, I advised you to turn off your television, computer, smartphone, tablet, and any other device that emits artificial light at least 1 hour before going to bed to improve your sleep. But according to the National Sleep Foundation, more than 90 percent of Americans use their electronic devices in the hour before they go to bed.

Having any such gadget in your bedroom is obviously a form of temptation that could interfere with sleep. However, the special kind of light emitted can also significantly tinker with your brain, reducing your levels of melatonin, the sleep hormone.[60] Any light at nighttime interferes with melatonin production, but the blue light waves produced by electronic devices (as well as many energy-efficient lightbulbs) are especially effective at suppressing melatonin production.[61] Televisions once used a fluorescent tube, which produced a light composed of several colors, but not much blue, to light the screen. But now computers, TVs, and other electronic gadgets use backlit light-emitting diodes (LEDs), which produce a blue light. In one study, college students who used a tablet for 2 hours a night were found to have reduced their levels of melatonin by about 23 percent.[62] You'll recall that the suppression of melatonin, which helps us fall asleep, is linked to obesity.

Block the Blue

In addition to not using your electronic devices close to bedtime, there are at least two other ways to limit your exposure to blue light. You can download a free software program that automatically adapts the display on your computer, iPad, or iPhone (but not your TV), making it a warm color at night and like sunlight during the day. Once you type in your zip code, the app f.lux (justgetflux.com) adjusts the color automatically at the appropriate time. Another option is to wear amber-tinted, blue-blocking goggles after sundown, which has been shown to counter melatonin suppression and improve sleep quality.[63] The glasses address not just the use of your electronic devices but also exposure from lightbulbs and other sources. You can find amber-lens goggles made by Uvex, Solar Shield, and others online—of course.

Need a Little Help Unplugging?

If your self-control can do with a little assist, check out the app Freedom (macfreedom.com), which works on both PCs and Macs. It allows you to block the Internet for up to 8 hours at a time. You could set it for 1 hour before your bedtime to avoid temptation when you should be getting ready to sleep, or use it just for your "unplugging" time. You can always reboot to get back online. Anti-social (anti-social.cc) is another program that blocks only social networking sites, so you can focus on work.

THE CELLPHONE CONUNDRUM

A recent survey found that 91 percent of adult Americans use a cellphone, and more than 38 percent of households have already cut the cord to a landline.[64, 65] At the beginning of 2014 there were an estimated 6.7 billion mobile phone users worldwide.[66] The smartphone is fast becoming the most commonly owned digital device, reaching 61 percent of all cellphone sales by 2013.[67] According to a 2014 online Google survey of 28,000 Canadian smartphone users, these users spend about 86 percent of their leisure time each day—about 7 hours!—watching its screen or the screen of another device.[68]

As anyone who has ever been late for a meeting or lunch date, run out of gas on a lonely road, or locked herself out of the house knows, life without a cellphone can be riskier, less convenient, and just plain messy. But you needn't have it on 24/7. All I'm asking is that you turn it off for 1 waking hour a day.

Your cellphone emits low levels of electromagnetic radiation, which your body can absorb. The International Agency for Research on Cancer, an arm of the World Health Organization, classifies cellphone radiation as "possibly carcinogenic." Almost 30 years of research has been inconclusive to date, but study is ongoing.[69] Nonetheless, we can take certain precautions to reduce our risk. (See "Cellphone Safety" on page 110.)

Cellphone Safety

In addition to installing a landline and using it when you're home to minimize cellphone use as much as possible, follow these guidelines:

- Use a hands-free headset, which can reduce radiofrequency (RF) energy eightfold.

- Don't wear your cellphone on your body when it's on.

- Earphone devices, such as Bluetooth, reduce RF energy, but be sure to remove them after use, as they continue to emit some radiation even when they're off.

- Text whenever possible to keep the phone away from your head.

- When reception is poor, resume the call later. The weaker the signal, the more radiation your phone emits as it strives to overcome poor reception.

- Only use a cellphone in a car if there is an external antenna.

If you're in the market for a new mobile, look for a model that emits lower levels of radiation than others.

UNDERACTIVE THYROID AND OVERWEIGHT

According to the National Cancer Institute, in recent decades the incidence of hypothyroidism (underactive thyroid), especially among women, has mushroomed. An underactive thyroid produces a lot less of the hormones T3 (triiodothyronine) and T4 (thyroxine), but more TSH (thyroid-stimulating hormone), created in an effort to restore the proper balance. Higher-than-normal TSH levels are a marker for hypothyroidism. Symptoms of the condition include depression, intolerance to cold, joint pain, and muscle cramps, along with fatigue and weight gain. It is also marked by a low resting metabolic rate, so it's not surprising that a sluggish thyroid can manifest as tiredness and obesity.

Israeli scientists have recently found changes in thyroid cells from healthy people after exposing them to electromagnetic fields (EMFs) similar to those emitted by cellphones.[70] This could indicate a connection between the rise in thyroid cancer cases and increased exposure to cellphone radiation. Irradiated thyroid cells multiplied at a significantly higher rate than non-irradiated cells in a control group. Other studies have shown changes in the saliva of frequent cellphone users that indicate higher levels of oxidative stress.[71] These preliminary studies raise more questions than they resolve, but are provocative.

A NIGHTTIME PARTNER, NOT

Many people sleep with their cellphone at their bedside. And the younger they are, the more likely they are to do so. Not a good idea. The very device that wakes you up in the morning may be keeping you up at night. The radiation emitted by cellphones can disrupt sleep. In addition to making it more difficult to nod off and experience long periods of deep sleep, radiation can cause headaches, confusion, and moodiness, according to a study that,

Cellphones and Thyroid Cancer: Is There a Connection?

There are concerns about a possible link between the dramatic increase in thyroid cancer in recent years and the increased amount of EMFs in our environment, in part due to a dramatic increase in cellphone use. According to the National Cancer Institute, thyroid cancer cases doubled between 1992 and 2012.[72] Although women are three times more prone to thyroid cancer, men in certain professions are also at high risk. It has been suggested that high rates among firefighters could be associated not with breathing carcinogens in smoke but instead with increased exposure to EMFs from their mobile two-way radio communication devices and the radio transmitters on fire engines.[73]

In 2009 the first study that explored the connection between cellphones and thyroid cancer looked at the levels of thyroid hormones in three groups of healthy college students: non-users of cellphones, moderate users, and heavy users.[74] Mobile users were found to have a statistically significant higher level of TSH and a slightly lower level of T4; T3 levels remained normal. The study authors wrote, "It may be concluded that possible deleterious effects of mobile microwaves . . . affects the levels of these hormones." Studies on rats indicate that exposure to EMFs can change the thyroid gland's structure and function.[75]

ironically, was funded by several mobile phone manufacturers.[76] About half the subjects participating in the study experienced such symptoms. The authors of the study noted that the radiation from a cellphone interferes with the ability to wind down and nod off.

In addition, if the device is right there, you'll probably feel the need to check out the latest beep, ring, or ping, and even return the call or respond to the text. That's borne out by a Swedish study that found a strong association between heavy mobile use by twentysomething adults and difficulties sleeping, as well as stress and depression.[77] I know that when I feel my phone vibrate, ring, or alert me to an e-mail, a text, a phone call, or a Twitter notification, it's, "Oh, gosh. What do I have to do?" Constantly being aware of these alerts is taxing. But when I turn off my cell, I can de-stress and regroup. Bottom line: Turn off your cellphone at night and don't use it as an alarm clock.

CELLPHONES AND WEIGHT— IT'S COMPLICATED

The association between cellphone use and obesity is less clear-cut than it is with television viewing. A study of Finnish teenage twins found a weak link between higher cellphone bills and higher BMI, in contrast to increased time at the computer, which was more straightforwardly related to higher BMI.[78] On the other hand, American college students who used their phones

Multiple Sources of "Electro-Pollution"

Cellphones aren't the only devices that emit electromagnetic radiation. The iPod in your briefcase or backpack, the GPS on your car dashboard, your computer and/or tablet, broadcast and mobile phone antennas, power lines, satellite TV, and the WiFi in your home and at Starbucks and the public library also all contribute to exposing us to 100 million times more EMFs than our grandparents experienced.[79] The difference is that we have more control over our exposure to our cellphones than we do to most of these other sources.

most frequently were found to be less physically active and less cardiovascularly fit than those who used their phones less.[80] The study's authors found that simply using the phone disrupts physical activity and can encourage sedentary behavior. Additionally, relatively high cellphone use is often a marker for other sedentary activities such as watching TV, playing video games, and using a computer.

The good news is that you can make a mobile phone live up to its name. Simply keep moving while you're talking, texting, or whatever. (Do be careful to watch your step.) Also, a number of phone apps—such as those that track activity, help you plan meals (or photograph them), or count calories—could help you manage your weight.

AVOID "TEXT NECK" TO STAND TALL AND LOOK SLIM

Using your cellphone incorrectly can pose a postural problem. Most people tilt their head to one side to hold the phone, which stretches the muscles on one side of their neck. Likewise, while texting, they thrust their neck forward, decreasing the curve of the neck and increasing the strain on it and the shoulders. This hunched posture even has a name: forward head posture. But I prefer the more recently coined term *text neck*. Over time, the posture stretches your trapezius muscles and shortens the muscles in the front of your neck, giving you a hunched-over appearance. You look like you have a belly, even if you don't. Remember, you want to stand tall with your shoulders down and your back straight to look as slim as possible.

Text neck is not confined to texting. If you're reading on a mobile device, your back hunch is probably even more extreme. Your head weighs about 10 pounds, but when you tilt your neck forward, it dramatically increases the pressure on your spine. If your mobile or tablet is in your lap, your neck is supporting what could feel like twice that weight or more.

Over time, chronic hunching can cause pinched nerves or even reverse the natural curve of your neck. In case you need frequent reminders to hold your cellphone at a proper angle (about 45 degrees), there's even a mobile app to help you avoid text neck (text-neck.com/text-neck-indicator—a-mobile-app.html). I know; it's ironic. If you hold your phone at a safe viewing angle, a green light shines in one corner of the device, but if the angle is bad, the light turns red. App aside, taking breaks every 20 minutes or so when using a computer or any mobile device is key to avoiding postural problems. Stand up, roll your shoulders and neck, or better yet, take a short walk to improve circulation.

Of course, text neck isn't the only postural issue. Thanks to our love affair with technology, sitting is at an all-time high, along with an epidemic of lower back injuries. And of course, when your back is killing you, you tend to exercise less, which makes it harder to slim down. Welcome to another vicious circle.

THE BEST TIME TO UNPLUG

Now that we've covered the pervasive influence of electronic devices, let's look at how to detach for 1 hour a day. There's actually no single time of day that works for everyone. Depending on your family responsibilities and work schedule, it could be first thing in the morning, around dinnertime, or before bed—whatever works for you. Consider these possibilities.

- **EARLY BIRDS.** While the rest of the household is still in the sack is a perfect time to meditate, pray, do breathing exercises, or write in your journal. If you want to be more active, try taking a walk or doing your resistance exercises. Exercising first thing means you're more likely to do it.[81, 82] If you're up early enough, you can watch the sun rise, always an inspiring experience. Or perhaps just having an hour to yourself for breakfast and catching up on your reading before the kids are up and clamoring for attention is your daily gift to yourself.

- **ALL IN THE FAMILY.** The tradition of the family dinner has declined in recent decades. Only 40 percent of families eat together several times a week. A study that reviewed 17 prior studies (of almost 18,300 kids and teens) found potent evidence of how important it is to sit down for dinner as a family.[83, 84] Kids who ate with their family at least three times a week were 12 percent less likely to be obese, 24 percent less likely to eat unhealthy foods, and 35 percent less likely to have an eating disorder. For teens, eating meals as a family frequently is also associated with doing better in school and being less likely to drink alcohol or take drugs.[85] All are great reasons to make your unplugged time the dinner hour.

If possible, involve older kids in planning the menu and making the meal, and allow them to drive the conversation at the table. Explain that you're turning off your phone, the TV, and any other devices while you're preparing and eating so you can all enjoy your meal together, tune out any distractions, and catch up on one another's day. It may be difficult to coordinate schedules to do this every night; 3 or 4 nights a week may be more realistic for those with school-age kids. Many parents find that their kids initially resist this idea, but come around to appreciating it and even inviting their friends to join them. Nor are kids the only ones to benefit. Mindful eating has been shown to reduce stress and prevent weight gain in overweight women without dieting.[86]

- **NIGHTTIME RITUAL.** The hour before bed is a natural time to unplug. By turning off all distractions, including screens that emit blue light, which interferes with melatonin production, you're more likely to naturally bridge the transition from waking activities to quality sleep time.

SWAP SIT TIME FOR FIT TIME

So what are you going to do with that time once you're untethered from your electronic devices? If it's not late in the evening, one obvious option is to get moving! Take that walk you promised yourself you would. (If you feel safer with your cellphone on your person, just turn it off.) It's a great opportunity to tune in to the natural world or resolve an issue you've been putting off. Or do your resistance exercises. You'll still have almost an hour for another activity. How about cleaning out that closet you've always wanted to attack or spending some quality time in your garden? The point is that this is your time to do anything you want, whether it's roughhousing with your kids or hopping on your bicycle.

You're not allowed to use a phone on the golf course, which is actually one of the reasons I took up golf. Until recently, I'd figured that golf takes too much time, and who has that time? Not me. I'd been using that excuse for years, and then I realized—wait a minute: That's the whole reason why I *should* golf. It's a great way to take time to unplug from the digital world and go on a mini mental vacation. Golf allows me to be active—I walk about 14,000 steps on an 18-hole course—and I'm also not using my phone, my computer, or the Internet during that time. It's a good example of how you can simultaneously accomplish two of the My 5 behaviors.

QUIET TIME

Assuming that you're already getting in your daily 10,000 steps and your resistance exercises, your unplugged hour needn't involve lots of physical exertion. Instead, you can pursue a new activity or one you'd put aside. Perhaps it's playing the piano or another instrument or building models, knitting, or painting watercolors. You might choose to read a magazine, do a crossword puzzle, take a bubble bath, or putter in your workshop. The only guideline is no TV, no radio, no Internet, etc. Free yourself from all that chatter and stimulation and you'll be amazed at how

Meditation Goes Mainstream

To many people, meditation conjures up images of gurus on mountaintops, chanting chakras, and new-age mysticism. Mindfulness meditation, on the other hand, is eminently practical. It can also withstand scientific scrutiny. In fact, Aetna and other health insurance companies and corporations such as General Mills have climbed on the mindfulness meditation bandwagon because it's a proven way to reduce stress, enhance productivity, and reduce certain health problems. For individuals, its simplicity enhances its appeal. All you need is a quiet place, your own breath, and perhaps a rolled-up blanket or a few pillows to get comfortable. For more on this practice, visit mindfulnessmeditationinstitute.org, emindful.com, or zencast.org.

de-stressed and refreshed you feel when you return to the hubbub of the contemporary world.

Another quiet way to spend your unplugged hour is to engage in mind-quieting practices. Meditation has been practiced for thousands of years in India, China, and other parts of the Far East, and for decades in the West. You may already meditate. The kind most often studied by scientists is mindfulness meditation or open-monitoring meditation, in which you simply pay attention to all the things happening around you without reacting. Mindfulness is a way of living in the moment and being nonjudgmental.

MEDITATION, STRESS REDUCTION, AND WEIGHT

Regular practice of mindfulness meditation reduces stress and instills calmness and focus.[87] It can also treat depression[88] and significantly reduce stress and anxiety.[89] High levels of cortisol are associated with stress, as well as with being overweight. Individuals who participated in an intensive 3-month retreat found a direct relationship between improved mindfulness meditation and lowered cortisol levels.[90] The practice also enhances immune response and increases brain activity.[91-93]

Mindfulness encourages self-awareness and enhances self-regulation, motivation, empathy, and social skills, all valuable aids in helping foster weight loss. Recently, a small study connected mindfulness with weight management.[94] Overweight women were divided into two groups, neither of which was following a weight-loss program. One group trained in stress management and practiced mindfulness meditation each day; the other group did not. The first group was able to reduce stress, as indicated by reduced cortisol levels, and reduce "comfort" eating; the other was not. Several other studies have shown greater self-control over overeating (or binge eating) after enrolling in mindfulness meditation groups.[95, 96]

I love this next study because it symbolizes what much of this book is about: Five groups of people were assigned to walk quickly or slowly, and some were told to meditate while they walked. They did so by simply counting their

Five Key Points in Chapter 5

1. Using most electronic devices involves sitting, which makes it more difficult to lose weight. Multiple devices and additional functions have dramatically increased the use of all devices, and along with it magnified inactivity.

2. Watching TV is associated with mindless overeating, poor food choices, and obesity. The more hours you watch, the heavier you're likely to be. You're also more apt to lose track of what you've eaten and eat more throughout the day. Cutting TV time has been shown to enhance weight-loss efforts.

3. Overuse or constant pinging of devices can result in stress and depression, which can lead to overeating. Social media use can also create anxiety. Depression, stress, and anxiety are all associated with overeating and obesity.

4. Blue light emitted by electronic devices can interfere with melatonin production and impair sleep, which is directly linked to weight gain.

5. A sluggish thyroid, which might be associated with increased exposure to electromagnetic fields of cellphones, slows the metabolism and often results in weight gain.

steps, repeating "one, two," as they walked. After 16 weeks, those who walked and meditated, regardless of the speed at which they walked, displayed the lowest levels of stress and the highest levels of mood enhancement.[97]

We've covered many bases in this chapter. Many of them have an effect on your weight; some address other health issues. All in all, I hope that the clear and possible impacts of our dependence on electronic devices will help strengthen your resolve to take a break from their intrusions. Once you get in the habit, as I have with my golf game mini vacations, you'll wonder how you managed without unplugged time.

In the next chapter, we'll get into the specifics of the diet component of My 5 so you can begin shedding those 5 pounds today. Before you know it, these simple and easy changes in your daily routine will deliver the results you're looking for.

PART

2

5 DAYS
5 POUNDS

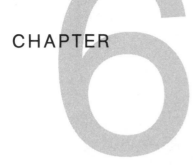

CHAPTER 6

THE 5-DAY DIET

Now that you've learned about all five components of the My 5 Plan, let's get cracking on shedding those 5 pounds. In Chapter 1, we discussed the proportions of protein, fibrous carbohydrates, and healthy fats that will make up your meals and team up to burn fat fast, as well as boost your energy. Now let's get into the specifics with a ground plan for the next 5 days, complete with meal plans, guidelines on portion sizes, snack suggestions, advice on how to get meals on the table, and some "convenience" foods to have on hand so you can always get a meal on the table, pronto. When you've finished this chapter, you'll truly understand how easy it is to eat this way throughout the day, no matter where you are.

If you're like many busy people, I suspect that you wind up eating at least some or perhaps many of your meals away from home. I certainly do. I travel a lot and often have to eat in restaurants or hotels. For many people who are watching their weight, this can spell trouble, but the vast majority of the foods you'll be eating on My 5 are readily available in your company cafeteria, the local deli, salad bar, or coffee shop, and certainly at most restaurants. The snacks are also easy to find and/or tote along in your purse or backpack.

In addition to being super simple, the diet part of My 5 is also versatile. That's why I'm giving you two options in each of the 5 days' worth of meal plans. Option 1 relies primarily on recipes that appear in Part 3. Option 2 includes items that are easy to find at a salad bar, restaurant, or deli, such as a turkey burger, Cobb salad, or a shrimp stir-fry, along with readily available snacks. Don't assume that just because an item appears on a menu that it's good to go. You may have to ask a few questions to find out exactly what's in any salad and make sure, for example, it's not drowning in high-fat, high-sugar salad dressing. The same applies to sandwiches: You won't want it if it comes on a huge white roll slathered with mayo. For more advice on eating out, see "Make Your Wishes Clear" below.

Make Your Wishes Clear

Here are strategies for ordering meals in a restaurant or deli during the first 5 days, along with suggestions to get what you actually want.

EGG DISHES: Ask for egg whites only or just one yolk cooked in a teaspoon of olive oil, and one piece of high-fiber bread on the side.

SALADS: Ask if the croutons, mozzarella, salami, or other high-fat or starchy carbs can be omitted, and request oil and vinegar on the side. You may have to remove any offending items yourself, but you can control the dressing situation.

SANDWICHES: Request an open-face sandwich on high-fiber bread. If that's not available, simply deconstruct it and eat it with a fork. Also tell the server to hold the mayo.

BURGERS: Ask if you can have it in a lettuce cup or on a single slice of high-fiber bread instead of on a bun. If not, deconstruct.

MAIN DISHES: Ask if the sauce can be omitted or served on the side. It may be full of butter and white flour. Inquire if the chicken, fish, or shellfish is breaded or batter-dipped. If so, see if it can be grilled or baked instead.

SOUP: Avoid chicken noodle soup and others heavy on the pasta. Instead, opt for a hearty fish chowder or gumbo, or beef or chicken vegetable soup. Pea and lentil soup are other options. Pass on the saltines and request a slice of high-fiber bread.

You can follow one of these two options to a T, or more likely combine suggestions from the two to suit your schedule and lifestyle. For example, you might always pick up breakfast on the way to work during the work-week but enjoy making breakfast on the weekends. Perhaps you routinely eat out at lunchtime but make a point of having dinner together as a family, even if it means relying wholly or partially on offerings from a salad bar or take-out place. Perhaps your Friday-night ritual is to dine out with your partner or friends. When it comes to snacks, feel free to substitute any of the snack suggestions on page 124 for those on the meal plans. Whatever your preferences, you'll find options that let you quickly pull together a meal or find a suitable (and delicious) alternative in a restaurant. By Day 6, after following these 5 days of meal plans, you'll be able to continue confidently on your own.

THE BIG THREE

As you now know, protein, fat, and fiber all produce some degree of satiety on their own. But when all three come together in a meal, they create a powerful synergy that allows you to eat less and shed weight quickly. Your breakfast, lunch, and dinner will be composed of what I call the "holy trinity of satiety":

   1. Protein

   2. Fibrous carbohydrates

   3. Healthy fats

Healthy fats may be an integral part of your protein—as with salmon, for example. Or you may dress a salad or vegetables with one of the preferred oils and lemon juice or vinegar.

Your morning and afternoon snack will both include:

   1. Fibrous carbohydrates

   2. Protein

HANDY PORTION CONTROL

How much you eat is as important as what you eat. Follow the portion guidelines provided below and you'll find it easy to consume the recommended 50 percent of your calories as carbohydrates, 30 percent as protein, and 20 percent as fat. Forget about weighing or measuring foods. Simply use your hand as a guide. Yes, big guys get to eat a larger portion than petite women. No surprises there!

MAIN MEALS:

- One portion of protein = a piece at least the mass of your whole hand

- One portion of either a high-fiber whole grain, a high-fiber fruit, or a high-fiber starchy vegetable = what fits in your palm

- One portion of healthy fats = one thumb (if not in protein source)

Pile on the produce: Have at least two fistfuls of nonstarchy vegetables—or as much as you wish.

Meals Made Simple

In Chapter 1, you learned about all the great foods you'll be eating, and now that you know how to judge portions, I'll show you how easy it is to turn them into three meals and two snacks a day. To make it really simple, I've come up with six types of speedy, scrumptious, slimming meals:

1. Smoothies   **4.** Salads

2. Scrambles   **5.** Soups

3. Sandwiches   **6.** Stir-Fries and Skillet Dishes

You'll find recipes for some options in each category, and they'll also turn up in the meal plans on the following pages. Remember, you're not limited to only these six categories as long as you're getting your protein, fiber, and healthy fats in the right proportions. And when eating in a Japanese restaurant, you'll find two more types of dishes that suit the My 5 Plan. Which brings me to my seventh and eighth favorite dishes: sushi and sashimi. Many supermarkets also offer take-out versions.

SNACKS:

- One portion of protein = at least the size of two thumbs

- One portion of either whole grains or fibrous carbohydrate = three thumbs

- However, nuts and seeds are much more calorically dense, so read the label to be sure a snack serving is close to 150 calories.

NOTE: In following the recipes (see page 173), the number of servings assumes a weight of 175 pounds or less. If you weigh more, increase the portion size for meals (but not snacks) by one-third.

A Perfectly Portable Snack

I'm big fan of jerky, a tasty and portable form of high-quality protein. Jerky harkens back centuries, when indigenous peoples used it as a way to preserve meat. The Incan name for dried meat is *ch'arki,* which later evolved into what we now call jerky. I like Oberto turkey and beef products because they contain no preservatives. If you're adventuresome, also look for salmon, buffalo, ostrich, and venison varieties of jerky.

WHAT'S ON THE SNACK MENU?

With snacks being such an important component of My 5, they must be tasty and filling, plus combine protein and fiber. The following suggestions cover all bases. Each contains roughly 150 calories and at least 5 grams of fiber and 5 grams of protein:

- Nonfat plain Greek yogurt with berries

- Celery with almond butter

- High-fiber crackers with sliced turkey

- Cut veggies with hummus

- Cut veggies with onion dip or ranch dip made with Greek yogurt

- Roasted soy nuts*

- Roasted chickpeas* (The Good Bean is a great brand)

- Jerky (all natural) with an apple

- Freeze-dried green peas*

- Apple with low-fat string cheese

- High-protein, high-fiber snack bars**

- Pear and sliced turkey breast

- Cucumber and smoked salmon

- Steamed edamame (green soybeans)*

- Air-popped popcorn* (5 cups)

- 1 cup high-protein, high-fiber cereal (Kashi GoLean)

Check out the meal plans starting on page 126 for more suggestions.

These foods contain both fibrous carbohydrates and protein.
**Bars and other packaged snacks must contain no more than 150 calories and at least 5 grams of fiber and 5 grams of protein.*

LOAD UP YOUR SHOPPING CART

You're probably chomping at the bit to rush right out to the supermarket so you can take your first steps in your journey to subtract 5 pounds. If you opt to follow Option 1 of the 5 days of meal plans that follow to the letter, simply create your shopping list from the ingredients you don't already have on hand. If you plan to swap out beef for chicken, for example, or Bibb lettuce for romaine, be sure to modify your list.

For other meals, with the following foods in the fridge, freezer, or pantry, you'll never find yourself in a situation where there's "nothing to eat."

- **PROTEIN:** Chicken or turkey breasts (skinned or remove skin before cooking) or non-breaded "tenders," ground turkey, eggs and/or cartons of separated egg whites, tuna or salmon (canned in water or vacuum-packed bags), shrimp (fresh, frozen, or canned). *Time-savers:* fully cooked fish fillets in individual-portion cook-in bags to pop in the oven, cooked turkey or chicken breast slices or chunks

- **DAIRY:** Low-fat or nonfat milk, cheese, cottage cheese, Greek yogurt (plain, unsweetened), and kefir (drinkable yogurt)

- **FIBROUS VEGETABLES:** Salad greens and garnishes and fresh, frozen, or canned veggies, canned lentils and other legumes, frozen edamame. *Time-saver:* trimmed and bagged veggies, washed and bagged salad mixes and coleslaw

- **FRUIT:** Apples, pears, citrus fruits, kiwis, and fresh or frozen berries. *Time-savers:* trimmed and cut-up fruits

- **WHOLE GRAINS:** Oatmeal (not instant), brown wild rice, quinoa, wheat berries, etc.; also high-fiber bread, tortillas, and crispbreads/crackers (see page 14).

- **SNACKS:** Popcorn (air popped); nuts; seeds; roasted soy nuts; chickpeas; frozen edamame; hummus; high-fiber, high-protein snack bars; and high-fiber, high-protein chips

- **HEALTHY FATS:** Olive oil, cooking spray, avocados, nut spreads, seeds

THE MEAL PLANS

DAY 1

	OPTION 1	OPTION 2
Breakfast	PB and Grape Smoothie (page 179)	Egg white scramble with avocado slices, 1 slice high-fiber toast, ½ grapefruit
AM Snack	Lite French Toast (page 207)	6 oz plain low-fat Greek yogurt with strawberries
Lunch	Mediterranean Lemon-Chicken Soup (page 200)	Spinach and mushroom salad topped with salmon and vinaigrette
PM Snack	Bell Pepper and Turkey Roll-Ups (page 208)	Hummus with carrot sticks
Dinner	Shrimp and Black Bean Stir-Fry (page 202)	Turkey burger on ½ high-fiber bun, string beans

No-Time-to-Cook Meals

If you're not really into cooking or simply don't have time on certain days, you can "assemble" a variety of lunches and dinners using prepared (cooked and sliced) ingredients from a good salad bar and/or deli. (With the exception of the eggs, you can also find canned or jarred versions of the protein foods.) Following the serving-size guidelines on page 123, mix and match, picking one food from each column. Remember, you can always have as many non-starchy veggies as you wish.

PROTEIN	NON-STARCHY FIBROUS VEGETABLES	HEALTHY FATS	STARCHY FIBROUS CARBS
Chicken or turkey	Spinach	Olive oil	Wild rice
Salmon	Romaine lettuce	Pumpkin seeds	Quinoa
Shrimp	Zucchini	Avocado	Raspberries
Hard-boiled eggs	Tomato	Nuts	Apple
Tofu	Bell peppers		High-fiber bread
Lentils/beans			Cucumber
Broccoli			

DAY 2

	OPTION 1	OPTION 2
Breakfast	Artichoke, Mushroom, and Smoked Salmon Scramble (page 181)	1 cup cooked oatmeal (not instant) with low-fat cottage cheese and berries
AM Snack	Nonfat cappuccino (or decaf nonfat cappuccino or tea with low-fat milk) and a pear	Apple with low-fat string cheese
Lunch	Grilled Cheese, Pear, and Turkey Sandwich (page 188)	Tuna (or smoked salmon) on tossed salad with vinaigrette
PM Snack	Red Lentil Puree (page 209)	Turkey jerky and bell pepper slices
Dinner	Saffron Shrimp Paella (page 203)	Chicken fajitas in a lettuce cup (no tortillas); hummus and 2 crispbreads

WHAT'S FOR BREAKFAST?

A scramble or smoothie always hits the spot. For a breakfast scramble, I might make a breakfast burrito. The protein comes from the egg whites, black beans, and cheese. Tomatoes, spinach, and beans provide the fibrous carbo-hydrates. I'll cook the scramble in a little olive oil for my healthy fat. There's also protein in the tortillas as well as some starchy fibrous carbohydrates. For a condiment, I'll sprinkle on some Tabasco or another hot sauce. With all the food groups covered, it's a great on-the-go breakfast. See how simple it is!

Smoothies are another speedy breakfast option, and can be a great way to get leafy greens into your morning meal. For example, the greens and fruit for the Apple, Peach, and Spinach Smoothie on page 180 provide your fibrous carbohy-drates. Protein powder and macadamia nuts supply the protein and healthy fats. Toss everything in the blender with a few ice cubes, and you have a delicious breakfast on the double. When ordering a smoothie in a restaurant, ask to have it made with unsweetened almond milk and plain low-fat Greek yogurt, along with a tablespoon of peanut butter to boost the protein, and your preferred fruits.

Other options include oatmeal (not the instant kind) served with steamed low-fat milk or cottage cheese and berries. Or have Kashi GoLean with low-fat milk and berries. Add some slivered almonds to up the protein content.

DAY 3

	OPTION 1	OPTION 2
Breakfast	Apple, Peach, and Spinach Smoothie (page 180)	3 hard-boiled eggs (use just 1 yolk), berries, and 1 slice high-fiber bread
AM Snack	Pear Crumble with Greek Yogurt (page 210)	Apple slices with almond butter
Lunch	Chopped Chicken and Pep-peroni Salad on Mixed Greens (page 194)	Chopped salad of lettuce, turkey, garbanzo beans, tomato, low-fat mozzarella, and tomato with vin-aigrette
PM Snack	Skinny Guacamole (page 211) with crackers	⅓ Hass avocado with a squeeze of lemon and chile flakes on a high-fiber cracker
Dinner	Manhattan-Style Chicken-Corn Chowder (page 198)	Baked salmon, small baked potato, sautéed spinach

ON THE LUNCH AND DINNER MENU

For a filling main-dish salad, check out my Chopped Chicken and Pepperoni Salad on Mixed Greens on page 194. The vegetables, which are a great source of fiber, are tossed with a vinaigrette made with that classic healthy fat, olive oil. Chicken breast, pepperoni, and chickpeas provide plenty of protein. On a cold day, a hearty soup like Creamy White Bean and Kale Soup on page 201 hits the spot. The beans and cheese offer up protein, while kale, tomatoes, and onion deliver the fibrous carbohydrates, and olive oil provides healthy fat. Serve with high-fiber bread for a starchy carbohydrate.

Sometimes only a sandwich will do the trick at lunchtime. How about the Charred Corn and Cumin Chicken Wrap on page 189? Chicken delivers the protein; tomatoes, onion, and red pepper the fibrous carbohydrates, along with a high-fiber tortilla. One of my favorite dinners is a shrimp stir-fry, such as the one on page 202. Shrimp, egg white, and black beans serve up the protein, the veggies and black beans provide the fiber, and sesame oil brings the healthy fat. A little brown rice adds some starchy carbs.

DAY 4

	OPTION 1	OPTION 2
Breakfast	Spinach Omelet with Feta and Avocado (page 182)	1½ cups Kashi GoLean cereal with low-fat milk, slivered almonds, and berries
AM Snack	Chocolate-Avocado Mousse with Raspberries (page 212)	½ cup plain low-fat Greek yogurt with cantaloupe cubes
Lunch	Spicy, Crunchy Wheat Berry Salad (page 192)	Cobb salad with vinaigrette
PM Snack	Turkey jerky and apple	Air-popped popcorn
Dinner	Saffron Shrimp Paella (page 203)	Shrimp and vegetable stir-fry with brown rice

DAY 5

	OPTION 1	OPTION 2
Breakfast	Italian Frittata with Zucchini, Leeks, and Parmesan (page 185)	Almond milk and Greek yogurt smoothie with 1 tablespoon peanut butter, strawberries, and ½ banana
AM Snack	Berry-Muesli Yogurt Parfait (page 213)	Container of plain low-fat Greek yogurt with 2 tablespoons All-Bran and berries
Lunch	Turkey, Barley, and Chard Soup (page 199)	Chicken-vegetable soup with high-fiber crackers
PM Snack	Air-popped popcorn with grated reduced-fat Parmesan cheese	Carrot sticks with ranch dip
Dinner	Korean Chicken Stir-Fry (page 204)	Grilled chicken breast; spinach and chickpea salad with vinaigrette

Now that you know how easy it is to put meals and snacks together, keep reading to take a closer look at the synergy inherent in the My 5 Plan.

CHAPTER 7

SAY YES TO SUCCESS

While I was writing this book, I was often asked what it's about. I'd answer that it's basically about five yes-or-no questions to ask yourself every night before you go to bed. To the extent that you're able to answer yes to all of them, you'll have optimized absolutely everything necessary to shed 5 pounds in as many days. That's the essence of the book—it's as simple as that. Success is answering yes to all five of these questions:

1. Did you eat three meals with protein, fibrous carbohydrates, and healthy fats, plus two snacks, today?
2. Did you do at least 5 minutes of resistance exercises today?
3. Did you take 10,000 steps today?
4. Did you sleep at least 7 continuous hours last night?
5. Did you unplug (no phone, TV, or computer) for at least 1 hour today?

At the end of the day, if you have five yes answers, pat yourself on the back. That's success. Success happens as a by-product of our successful actions. Your primary goal shouldn't be a number on the scale, because we don't have direct control over that number. (Remember, the scale doesn't necessarily tell the truth, or at least the whole truth.) Our actions provide indirect control, of course. If you've shed 5 pounds, you've probably succeeded in making those five behaviors your goals—and in achieving them. Losing weight, feeling better, and looking better are desirable, but they're all *by-products* of success that come from fulfilling those five daily behaviors. As psychologist Viktor Frankl wrote, "Make the process your goal. You cannot pursue success, for success, like happiness, can only ensue and does so as the natural byproduct of dedicating yourself to a process."

If you do less of one of the five essential behaviors, you can't really compensate by doing more of the other things. For example, upping your activity from 10,000 steps to 20,000 steps a day is terrific, but it won't make up for not getting enough sleep, overeating, or skipping out on your resistance training.

I've been using My 5 with my private clients for a few years now. They love the simplicity of it. It's easy to understand. It's not just a diet. I'm basically asking them to keep track of themselves. Knowing that they have to report to me is helpful at the beginning. But inevitably, when they're not happy with their weight, or something is off, they'll look within and say, "Well, let me look at my yes's or no's over the past few days, and it will be obvious what I'm not doing enough of."

People get frustrated when they're not seeing results, and it can be hard for them to gauge why that's the case, particularly when the goals are qualitative, such as eating healthy or becoming fitter. But with the My 5 approach, it's very easy to know how you're doing because all five behaviors are quantifiable, measurable, tangible, and immediate. It's all very black and white. You can immediately ascertain your results based on your responses to the questions.

Think of it this way. If your car isn't running properly, you get a technical diagnosis to find the root of the problem. You bring your car into the garage, and the mechanic plugs it into the computer to see empirically what's wrong. And it's no different with your body, except the diagnosis is so simple you don't need a computer. Or an expert. Just answering the five questions will tell you what's wrong if you're not feeling good—or good about yourself.

THE SYNERGY OF FIVE

In the Introduction, I mentioned the *gestalt* inherent in the My 5 Plan. In plain English, each of the five behaviors works synergistically with the others to become more than the sum of its parts. The beauty of My 5 is that none of the behavior changes requires a significant amount of time. For the most part, they're all things you're already doing, although you may need to make some adjustments. They complement and amplify each other. For example, if you're sleeping better, you'll have more energy to hit your goal of 10,000 steps a day plus do your 5 minutes of resistance exercises. Conversely, if you hit your 10,000 steps and complete your resistance exercises, you'll most likely sleep better.[1] When you get 7 or 8 hours of rest, you're going to make better eating choices. In the process of taking 10,000 steps a day, you'll almost certainly be unplugging from technology more. And so on. It's all connected.

Synergy pays dividends. In one study, more than 400 overweight or obese sedentary women were assigned to one of four groups and told to either engage in 45 minutes of moderate-intensity exercise 5 days a week; follow a reduced-calorie, low-fat diet; combine the same exercise and diet recommendations; or make no changes in behavior. After a year, the exercise-only group lost an average of 4.4 pounds, and the diet-only group an average of 15.8 pounds.[2] But the women who combined exercise and diet lost almost 20 pounds. Moreover, two-thirds of the women in that group had achieved the study goal of losing 10 percent of their initial weight.

Can You Laugh Off the Pounds?

Some people self-medicate with food to sooth negative emotions, but how about another way to neutralize those feelings and simultaneously break the impulse to overeat? Laughing decreases the amount of cortisol, epinephrine, and growth hormone, among other factors, which reduces stress.[3, 4] Since stress can trigger overeating, theoretically laughter can help weight-loss efforts, but until recently there was no evidence of this. Now there is. In a recent study, people watched video clips that were more or less likely to elicit laughter while they were hooked up to monitors. When the subjects laughed, their energy expenditure and heart rate levels rose by 10 to 20 percent above resting levels.[5] Hey, it's not much, but every little bit counts.

AN ENTWINED ROPE

Here's another way to envision the *gestalt* of My 5. Each of the five behaviors described in the previous chapters is in and of itself like a rope that will support you and give you strength. But when you intertwine these five ropes, they become like the giant anchor rope that a tugboat uses to tow an ocean liner out to sea. Should one of those five ropes weaken and break, the other four are strong enough to hold everything together. The four ropes may not be able to hold the load indefinitely, because inevitably there will be more pressure on each of them, but they can do the job for a while until the fifth rope can be repaired or replaced. Think of My 5 as that giant intertwined rope.

Now, each one of those smaller entwined ropes that make up the big rope has many strands—which reminds me of a Spanish proverb: "Habits are at first cobwebs, then cables." For example, one of the smaller ropes is good nutrition, which in turn is composed of interwoven strands such as enough protein, fiber, healthy fats, and adequate hydration. The strands that make up the sleep rope include a minimum number of hours of shut-eye, good-quality sleep, a quiet environment, and darkness. Did you have caffeine just before you went to bed? Did you eat a big meal late at night? Do you have indigestion? Are you at the mercy of your bladder? Each one of those strands is represented by the answer to these questions and impacts the strength of the sleep rope. With exercise, the 5 minutes of resistance exercise a day is the rope, and the strands are the individual exercises that address all the main muscle groups, as well as the intensity with which you're training and the variation you introduce by changing the number of sets and reps of the various exercises. The same applies to the ropes of aerobic activity and tuning out for an hour a day.

FIVE FOR FIVE

Let's return to the five questions. If the answer to any single question is in the negative, the result sets off a whole cascade of effects. Say you don't eat five times nicely spaced across the day. You'll be hungrier. You might burn lean muscle tissue instead of body fat for energy. Perhaps you'll be too tired to do your resistance exercise. I'm not saying that you shouldn't walk 20,000 steps a day, but if you do, don't kid yourself that it gives you an excuse to stay up half the night or have a chocolate chip muffin and a couple of glasses of wine every day. Following four of the behaviors I recommend but ignoring the fifth doesn't make things right.

If you decide to run 2 hours a day, every single day, and eat only 800 calories a day, it's simply not sustainable. You won't be happy and the results you're looking for will elude you. But make several relatively modest changes in your behavior, all of which are eminently doable and which develop a powerful synergy, and you'll find it increasingly easy to answer yes to each question at the end of the day.

AIM FOR SIMPLICITY, EFFICIENCY, AND SAFETY

That said, don't beat yourself up if one day you don't answer all five question with a yes. There's no failure on this program. There's simply another moment in which you can turn things around and begin doing the right things. That brings up another point: I have clients who come to me and say, "Guess what? I'm going to start a hard-core weight-loss program. I'm going to stop smoking and being sedentary. And I'm going to start running an hour a day, do another hour of weight training, and start meditating." So they do begin all those things, and after 2 weeks they say, "Oh, my gosh, I got through it! I feel like a different person. I lost 6 pounds, and I have clarity. So now what do I do?"

At that point, I say, "Okay, do what I told you to do 2 weeks ago. Eat protein and fibrous carbohydrates five times a day, get at least seven hours of sleep, take 10,000 steps a day," and so on. Their response usually is, "Well, if I'd started that 2 weeks ago, how much weight would I have lost?" I tell them that it would probably be the same 6 pounds. They answer, "You mean I didn't need to do all that stuff?" The point is that there are different ways to get to the same result. I always believe in taking the path of least resistance. And that path is the simplest, the most efficient, and the safest way. And that's what this book is all about.

TOMORROW IS ANOTHER DAY

The reality is that some days we don't achieve all five behaviors. As the old saying goes, life happens. I have a newborn baby at home. She wakes up every 2 or 3 hours to let us know that she's hungry. Needless to say, my sleep is severely compromised, and I have to struggle to get in my 7 to 8 hours of continuous sleep. What do you do in a situation like this, which is out of your control? In my case, I make an added effort to be sure I definitely stay on top of the other four behaviors, which are within my control. Because I'm still hitting four out of five, I'm still making progress. So when my sleep patterns return to normal—I'm counting the seconds!—my habits will still be my habits.

Another strategy that can come in handy on days when you aren't able to answer yes to every question is to ask yourself, "Where was I when I started?"

If you were zero for five then, and now you're three for five, you're definitely moving in the right direction. Feel good about what you've accomplished today and be optimistic that your results will keep getting better as you add another behavior to your day.

It's inevitable that there will be times when we're unable to complete one or more behaviors. Recently, I flew to see a client on the other side of the world. The trip took 21 hours, crossing the international date line, so I actually arrived nearly 2 days after I'd departed! Needless to say, I didn't walk my 10,000 steps, get my 7 to 8 hours of hours of sleep, or do my resistance exercise on the plane. I did manage to eat three healthy meals and two snacks, and of course, to unplug. Once in a while these days happen. Whether it's caused by a flight or the flu, sometimes we just cannot knock all five balls out of the park. It's out of our control.

That's okay. If you're five for five for 20 straight days, and then you're hit with one of *those* days, your rope is still strong. Each day you managed to go five for five is yet another strand woven into your rope. Its strength means that an occasional day when you cannot meet your goals won't do any significant harm.

TIME IS OF THE ESSENCE

Now let's deal with the monster hiding under the bed. Are you saying to yourself, "I'm so busy as it is, I can barely get through the day. How can you expect me to do all five of these things too?" Aha, the key word is *too*. Aside from the 5 minutes of resistance exercise, I'm not asking for any time out of your day. It doesn't take extra time to make better choices. You already sleep, but perhaps not long enough and not too well. You already eat, but perhaps not the right foods in the right proportions or at the right times. You already walk, of course, but probably not enough.

I'm *not* asking you to take precious minutes to drive to the gym (10 to 30 minutes); park, change, work out, and shower (60 to 90 minutes); and drive home (another 10 to 30 minutes). I'm *not* asking you to run a marathon or suffer through a spin class. And unless you never spend any leisure time in front of the TV or another electronic device, I'm only asking that you give yourself the gift of an hour to unplug and unwind. You'll actually gain an hour to enhance your own well-being. I'm *not* asking you to cook elaborate meals that no one else in the family will want to eat. The bottom line is that following My 5 is not about doing *more*; rather, it's about doing things smarter. It's simply another way of doing things, of making different choices.

THE ART OF PRIORITIZING

Many years ago I took a seminar on time management with Stephen Covey, author of *The 7 Habits of Highly Effective People*. The takeaway was that rather than focusing on what's urgent, we should prioritize what's important—the things that are dear to your heart and improve the quality of your life. As Covey put it, "The key lies in escaping the tyranny of the clock and following your internal compass." He also made a very interesting point: that when you're living according to your principles, your journey and your destination are the same. That applies perfectly to My 5. The behaviors that I'm asking you to embrace by saying yes to the five questions are not just about becoming 5 pounds slimmer in 5 days; they're also the same behaviors that can become an integral part of your life and therefore part of your life's journey.

Most of us are caught in a trap of wanting to do all sorts of things, but at the end of the day, the end of the week, or the end of the year, we invariably come up short. There's simply never the time to do those interesting things and achieve these admirable goals. This is a clock- or calendar-driven approach to achieving goals. But when you prioritize the things that really matter to you and get them done first, you set your own compass. So if you prioritize being slim, fit, well rested, and happy with yourself, you're going to arrange your days and your life to find the time for the five behaviors I recommend.

WRITE IT DOWN

Keeping a daily journal of your thoughts as well as your actions—the answers to the five daily questions—allows you to reflect on what you accomplished, what remains undone, and how you might do things differently in the future. Journaling makes you accountable, but only to yourself. Your memory is imperfect, but a journal isn't subject to forgetfulness. It's all

Five Ways to Use Your Time Well

Inherent in time management is planning ahead, so you don't find yourself halfway through the day with nothing ticked off your to-do list. Some helpful hints to take control:

1. PRIORITIZE WHAT'S IMPORTANT TO YOU. If you can't seem to find the time to take a half-hour walk but are wiling away hours on Facebook (or whatever), ask yourself if you're effectively making a decision that undermines your larger objective.

2. CREATE A SCHEDULE. Enter activities that matter most to you as you would any important event. It may seem odd to enter in your calendar items such as "do resistance exercises," "turn off TV," "have morning snack," etc., but by recording them, you're making it clear that they're as important as meeting a pal for lunch, seeing your accountant, and keeping other appointments.

3. SET SPECIFIC GOALS. By purchasing this book, you've set yourself a goal of losing 5 pounds in 5 days. Being specific about not just the goal but also in quantifying how and when you'll achieve it will mightily increase your likelihood of success.

4. PREPARE AND REVIEW. Take a few minutes in the morning to preview your day, deciding what you'll do and when to do it. In the evening, review your day to see what you achieved. By answering the five questions I've posed to you before you go to bed, you're doing just that.

5. LEARN TO SAY NO. All too often we agree to do something we really would prefer not to because we don't want to seem selfish. But accepting a task and resenting it is hardly a recipe for a job well done. If you truly don't have the time to do something and know it will interfere with doing what matters more to you, be forthright about it. Explain that you'd be happy to help out another time but right now you couldn't give it the attention it deserves.

there in black and white. Remember, your journal is for your eyes only, so be honest. It will take you only a few minutes a day to answer the five questions and make entries in the journal. By documenting your new behaviors—and if and when you occasionally depart from them, and what roadblocks got in the way—you'll begin to see patterns emerge.

Journal keepers have repeatedly been shown to be more successful at making permanent changes in their lives, and specifically in losing weight and keeping it off, than people who don't keep such a record. For example, in one study, almost 1,700 overweight or obese individuals were told to keep a food journal over a 6-month period. One of the most powerful predictors of weight-loss success was how many days an individual recorded his or her food intake in the journal.[6] People who did so 6 days a week lost, on average, significantly more weight as those who did so only 1 day a week or less.

I've provided journal pages for 5 days, starting on page 243, as well as a template you can copy for ongoing use.

IT'S NOT ABOUT WILLPOWER

When I talk to new clients who've tried various weight-loss programs without success or who've gained back weight (and often then some) after dieting, the issue of willpower inevitably comes up. They'll say something along these lines: "I really try to keep my appetite under control, but I'm so hungry my good intentions fly out the window." Or, "I'm fine until I sit down to eat, but then I'm so ravenous I can't stop eating." Or, "I know I should eat 'healthy' food but I crave junk food when I'm stressed, and I'm stressed much of the time."

If these scenarios resonate with you, you'll be happy to hear that willpower isn't an issue on My 5, thanks to eating three meals and two snacks spaced roughly 3 hours apart. You'll feel full all day without the blood sugar fluctuations that could lead to energy crashes and cravings. As long as you eat enough protein, fiber, and healthy fats, the appetite monster is kept at bay. And the 7-plus hours of sleep you'll be getting should keep the hormones ghrelin and leptin in balance, which also helps moderate your appetite. And when you feel satiated, you're also less vulnerable to making poor eating decisions.

FASTER IS BETTER

Now here's some really good news about initial rapid weight loss—and with it the premise of this book. Conventional wisdom says that it's easy to lose weight but hard to maintain that loss. Sadly, that's true. Conventional wisdom has also decreed that losing weight more slowly is more likely to result in permanent weight loss. I'm delighted to report that isn't true. Losing a good amount of weight quickly from the get-go is actually one of the predictors of successfully maintaining weight loss. In a review study, researchers found that the more pounds lost quickly, the more likely that weight loss would be maintained for at least 6 months.[7] According to this study, other factors also predicting successful weight-loss maintenance are being physically active, eating breakfast, and eating meals on a schedule—all integral to My 5 along with a number of psychological motivators.

Make It a Team Effort

Many self-help books will tell you that verbalizing your goal to others will increase your likelihood of success. I beg to differ. That strategy is basically about doing something because you'll be embarrassed if your friends and associates see that you didn't follow through. Actions speak louder than words. Instead of declaring your intention with words, declare it with your behaviors. It's the same as "do as I do, not as I say." I've seen this over and over again. When friends and family see a positive change in you, they want to know what you're doing and how to do it too. Lead by example and then you can eat similar meals, eat at the same time, take some of your steps together, and do things together while you unplug. Not surprisingly, people who follow a weight-loss program with friends, family, or coworkers achieve better results. One study found that people who wanted to lose weight who had at least one successful exercise buddy lost more weight than those who didn't have such a buddy.[8]

Another review study finds that initial weight loss is associated with long-term maintenance of lost weight, as long as people make lifestyle changes in diet, increased physical activity, and other behaviors. Again, My 5 hits all these bases and is designed to be an ongoing lifestyle.[9] The authors of this Swedish study write, "In conclusion, we find evidence to suggest that a greater initial weight loss as the first step of a weight management programme may result in improved sustained weight maintenance."

A more recent study adds fuel to the "faster is better for long-term weight loss" argument. The study put more than 260 middle-age obese women on one of three weight-loss programs of varying calorie content designed to achieve fast, moderate, or slow weight loss.[10] After a month, the women in the fast weight-loss group lost almost 2 pounds a week, compared with more than half a pound for the moderate weight-loss group and less than half a pound in the slow weight-loss group. Weight was checked again at 6 and 18 months. Women in the fast group were almost five times as likely to have lost 10 percent of their original weight and to have maintained that loss than the women in the slow group; those in the moderate group were three times as likely to have done so. The authors concluded, "Our study provides further evidence that . . . losing weight at a fast initial rate leads to greater short-term weight reductions, does not result in increased susceptibility to weight regain, and is associated with larger weight losses and overall long-term success in weight management."

A QUESTION OF MOTIVATION

I've always said that I don't need to motivate people. I fact, I believe that it's not possible for anyone else to motivate another person to take care of his or her health and body. If that sounds negative, that's the last thing I want to suggest. That's because I believe that people are *already* motivated. Everyone wants to look better, feel better, and perform better. Sometimes we forget that. Take a photo of yourself. Don't pose. Don't flex your muscles. Now take an honest look at your picture. Are you completely satisfied with what you see? What do you want to change? Now change it!

Don't feel bad about this. It's human nature to always want to improve yourself. I (still) occasionally eat more chocolate chip cookies than I should. And it bothers me that I'm not as lean as I was in my bodybuilding days. But the moment I wrote these two things down, I reminded myself of my motivation to do my five behaviors.

In the next chapter, we'll move beyond the 5 days to the rest of your life.

Five Key Points in Chapter 7

1. By asking yourself five questions each day, you track your behavior. Regularly having five yes answers means you're succeeding. It's a quantifiable, tangible, and immediate way to ascertain your results, and to self-diagnose when they aren't what you'd like.

2. Each of the five behaviors complements and amplifies the others to become more than the sum of their parts.

3. None of the behavior changes require a significant amount of time. You're already doing most of them, although you may need to make some adjustments.

4. On days when you aren't able to answer yes to every question, feel good about what you did accomplish that day and be optimistic that your results will keep getting better. And when you can't complete one or two of the behaviors—if you're sick or on a long plane trip, perhaps—don't let that be an excuse to not do the others.

5. Lead by example. When people see you changing your behavior and getting great results, they'll want to join the My 5 team.

CHAPTER

8

MY 5 FOR LIFE

As I explained in the last chapter, this book—and succeeding on My 5—is about answering yes to five questions every day. One question may not be on my list, but I suspect it's on your mind: "Have I lost 5 pounds?" Only you can answer that, but I'm confident that if you have answered the other five questions with a yes for the last 5 days, this one will be a yes as well. This book is about losing 5 pounds in 5 days, as the title declares loud and strong, but the subplot presents a way of being that promotes good nutrition, fitness, a healthy weight, and a feeling of mastery and accomplishment. Once you've experienced the powerful results you can achieve in a mere 5 days, you'll want to turn these behaviors into lifelong habits—and perhaps to continue losing weight.

If you're now on Day 6, congratulations on answering yes to the five questions over the last 5 days. Second, congratulations on optimizing your weight-loss journey with the five behaviors. You've taken the most important and effective steps that you possibly could to lose those first (or last) 5 pounds.

Isn't it amazing how much better you look and feel after just 5 days? (If you haven't yet started My 5 or haven't completed the first 5 days, well, you're getting a peek at my larger agenda!)

Now, imagine that you can feel even better, even fitter, and even slimmer. Yes, you can go from good to great, from striving to thriving, by making these new behaviors integral to your lifestyle. Now that you know how to do My 5, you can prove that practice really does make perfect. In this chapter, we'll talk about how to tweak things, whether your new objective is to ensure that those 5 pounds never return, to shed some more pesky pounds, or just to feel totally alive and in touch with your body.

So what do you on Day 6 and beyond? The simple answer is that you'll continue to do pretty much the same thing you've been doing over the past 5 days. However, you'll also make a few significant modifications.

- Now that you're getting at least 7 hours of sleep, aim for 8, if possible. Also follow the suggestions for improving the quality of your sleep.

- Consider unplugging from electronic devices for more than just 1 hour a day. And how about beginning mindfulness meditation, yoga, or another mind-calming practice for some or all of this time if you haven't already.

- Continue to eat foods composed of protein, fibrous carbohydrates, and healthy fats in three meals and two snacks a day, plus enjoy some small but pleasurable changes, which I'll tell you about shortly.

- Do your resistance exercises daily, although as you become fitter and stronger, you'll take things up a notch, as we'll discuss.

- Gradually up your daily steps beyond the minimum of 10,000.

THE SCALE DOESN'T LIE, OR DOES IT?

Careful readers will have noticed that never once have I told you to get on the scale. That's intentional. I know those 5 pounds are important to you, so you've probably weighed yourself at least once if not daily over the past 5 days. But now I'm suggesting that if you choose to weigh yourself, you do so at most *once a month*. Yes, once a month. Huh? "I thought this was a book about weight loss," you may be muttering. It is, but banishing excess pounds isn't the only part of this lifestyle. And weighing yourself daily or even weekly can actually be a deterrent to achieving your desired weight if the number on the scale upsets you rather than motivates you. Moreover, even the most advanced scale simply doesn't provide valid information.

For most of us, our weight fluctuates within a range of four (or even more) pounds on a daily (or even hourly) basis, depending on all your bodily functions. Your body's fluid level depends not just on when and how much you drank recently, or how much you're perspiring, but also on how much fluid you're retaining at any time. Premenopausal women are particularly subject to fluid retention at certain times of the month, causing weight fluctuation. As a result, you can't weigh yourself today and compare it with your weight 5 days later with any degree of accuracy, because you'll be a different point in your hormonal cycle.

On the other hand, if you weigh in once a month at the same time of day, you'll have a much more accurate gauge of whether you're continuing to lose— or maintaining your desired weight. A lot of my clients use the Fitbit Aria Wi-Fi Smart Scale. I like that I can keep track of the frequency that they're weighing themselves and make sure that they aren't getting on the scale too often. It collects data and also attaches the data to your activity level and your intake and graphs it. So it's a great way to keep track of all these things.

Another reason to hop on the scale just once a month is that you already have a perfectly good, immediate, and tangible way to measure your results. That's right: your yes answers to the five daily questions. I suspect that you can also tell whether you've dropped (or added) pounds just by the way your clothes—maybe some formerly snug jeans—fit. Nonetheless, weighing yourself *regularly* is an excellent motivational tool. Three-quarters of registrants in the National Weight Control Registry, all of whom have lost a minimum of 30 pounds and kept it off for a least a year, report weighing in regularly to keep those lost pounds at bay.[1]

MORE TO LOSE?

Whether or not you still have some pounds to shed after 5 days, you'll continue to follow the program as you have been. Meals and snack portions will remain relatively constant. There is one potential difference between those who are still slimming down and "maintainers," however, in terms of food intake. For both men and women, if your initial weight was more than 175 pounds, if and when it falls below that, you'll cut back on your intake slightly. Remember, you don't have to count calories, but by reducing portion sizes, you'll be coming down from about 1,600 to 1,700 calories to about 1,300 to 1,400 calories a day. Reminder: The recipes, starting on page 173, are designed for the lower intake level. (Increase portions by one-third as long as you weigh more than 175.) Also be prepared for the fact that as you get closer to your ideal body weight, the rate at which unwanted pounds disappear will slow. Typically, your appetite increases slightly at what's called your set point, the weight your body "wants" to be. That's perfectly normal and to be expected.

ADD SOME CULINARY VARIETY

Starting on Day 6, whether you're continuing to lose or maintaining your weight, your meals will still be composed of protein, fibrous carbohydrates, and healthy fats. However, variety is important on any eating plan, so I suggest you begin to try one new food a week. Perhaps it's a grain such as farro, quinoa, Kamut, or buckwheat (kasha). There's also an enormous world of fibrous vegetables out there. Broaden your salad choices to include watercress, arugula, kale, endive, or even baby bok choy. Remember, you can eat as many non-starchy vegetables you want, so feel free to serve more than one kind at a meal. Bored with spinach? Swap it for Swiss chard. Stuff red bell peppers, instead of the usual green ones, with ground turkey or beef. Rather than green cabbage, experiment with Chinese, savoy, napa, or red cabbage varieties. Many of these veggies are available frozen as well as fresh.

More Reasons to Add Variety to Your Diet

No foods are forbidden on My 5, although you'll continue to moderate your intake of starchy and sweet carbohydrates. On the other hand, weight-loss programs that limit the variety of foods, such as very low-carbohydrate diets, have a high dropout rate. That's because most people find them unsustainable. It's difficult to continue denying yourself certain foods indefinitely. There are also plenty of other reasons to eat a variety of foods:

- You're more likely to get all the vitamins, minerals, and other micronutrients necessary for good health.
- Using multiple ingredients in a soup or salad makes it seem more satisfying, so you eat less.
- You can experience how other cultures with low obesity rates eat.
- It facilitates eating out at restaurants.

When it comes to protein choices, expand beyond conventional meats to try bison, venison, and ostrich, all of which are increasingly available and boast a low fat content. Lentils and garbanzos are just the tip of the legume iceberg. Explore black-eyed peas and cannellini, fava, pinto, and pigeon beans, for starters. All are available canned and some can be found in the frozen food section.

While you're at it, how about trying a new recipe each week? Variety is truly the spice of life. My other books, *The 5-Factor Diet, The 5-Factor World Diet,* and *The Body Reset Diet* are packed with great recipes for you to try, in addition to the ones starting on page 173. (You can also order *The Body Reset Cookbook* from amazon.ca.)

TREAT YOURSELF (OCCASIONALLY)

My thinking about weight-loss dieting has evolved over the years. I used to recommend a weekly "cheat day" or "free day," meaning after 6 days on the program, you could take a day off. I still believe that it's important to enjoy an occasional treat. Feeling deprived has sabotaged many a restrictive diet. After being "good" for weeks on end, the urge to eat something forbidden gets the better of you. Once nothing is forbidden—okay, I really don't want you eating trans fats—there's less of an impulse to "cheat."

My revised dietary philosophy allows *two free meals a week*. Starting on Day 6, you get to pick when to have these meals or snacks—perhaps one on the weekend when you're out to dinner with friends or when you join your work buddies for lunch at the local pizza parlor. Or maybe you'll have a slice of birthday cake at a friend's party. In addition to the social aspects of not having to avoid certain types of food or restaurants, it's easier on your system to take two meal or snack "breaks" over the course of the week rather than have to transition back at the start of each week after a whole day "on break." In a study of participants in the National Weight Control Registry, those who reported eating consistently throughout the week were more successful at maintaining their weight loss than those who adhered to their diet more strictly during the week and eased off on the weekends.[2]

Interestingly, many of my clients have told me that since they now know that they can treat themselves occasionally, they're actually less inclined to do so, happily opting for a piece of fruit, for example, rather than a brownie, when they want something sweet.

MOVE MORE

Study after study confirms that people who are most successful at keeping off lost weight are those who are the most active and engage in exercise regularly, including those who have registered on the National Weight Control Registry. RealAge.com, which assesses your "real" age in terms of how your body is aging, claims that taking at least 10,000 steps a day is the equivalent of subtracting 4.6 years from your chronological age for women and 4.1 for men.[3]

Are you ready to go to the next level in terms of aerobic activity? Assuming you took at least 10,000 steps a day for the last 5 days, it's time to start inching up week by week. Starting in Week 2, add a minimum of 250 daily steps, taking your new goal to 10,250 steps. It's a baby step in the right direction. Do this every day for a week, and the following week, take it up to 10,500 steps—and so on. Or, if you've found it easy to log 10,000 steps, you can certainly go up in weekly increments of 500 daily steps. Ideally, you'll go up 1,000 steps daily per week. My wife and I aim for 14,000 steps a day. As always, it's better to go slowly and stay with it than to set your sights too high. Do what you can and keep pushing yourself. Numero uno: Listen to your body.

Once you've increased the number of steps, or even simultaneously, you can begin to increase aerobic intensity in one or more other ways:

- Increase your pace.

- Walk up stairs.

- Walk on an incline.

- Run or jog.

- Intersperse sprinting with walking or jogging.

SPEED UP

An obvious way to increase your aerobic activity is to pick up the pace. There are several ways to accomplish this.

- **WALK FASTER.** Brisk walking, meaning a speed of about 4 miles an hour, clearly burns more calories and increases oxygen intake more than a 2-miles-an-hour stroll. Gradually build up your speed by increasing the pace for a minute or two, reverting to your accustomed rate for 5 minutes, and so on. Over time, increase the length of the faster-walking periods until you're maintaining that rate overall. Compared with jogging, faster walking is easier on the hips and knees and diminishes the risk of injury.

- **RUN OR JOG.** Jogging isn't the best choice for everyone. Unlike brisk walking and running, which are more horizontal in nature and therefore not as likely to jar your torso, jogging involves moving your body up and down, which taxes your joints more. For some people, if done too long or too often, it can lead to injury. On the other hand, if you like to jog, be sure to wear shoes that give you the right support. If you're a runner, feel free to continue and/or blend it with walking.

- **SPRINT.** Short bursts of fast running burn the most calories of all these activities. A combination of sprinting and walking is even more effective than jogging. Like walking, sprinting is more likely to encourage good posture than jogging. Sprint interval training is a subcategory of high-intensity interval training (HIIT), which alternates low-intensity (walking or jogging) and high-intensity (sprinting) aerobic activity. As you get stronger and fitter, you can try a single 30-second burst a day, then two bursts a day, and finally three a day. Then you can increase the bursts to 45 seconds and later 60 seconds long. Always warm up before sprinting by taking a short walk or run. Again, listen to your body.

THE POWER OF SPRINTS

Numerous studies support the effectiveness of alternating sprints with moderately intense aerobic activity. A 2011 study at Bath University found that, remarkably, a mere 40 seconds of intense activity could make a difference.[4] Yes, just 40 seconds! Fifteen healthy but sedentary young adults followed a 6-week program called REHIT (reduced exertion high-intensity training), while a control group of 14 subjects did no exercise. The first week, the subjects bicycled gently for a couple of minutes, followed by a 10-second burst of intense cycling and then 2 minutes of cooldown. For the next 2 weeks, each session included a warmup, 15 seconds of sprinting, and 2 minutes of recovery, followed by another 15 seconds of sprinting, and concluded with a cooldown. In the next 3 weeks, two 20-second sprints were separated by 2 minutes of recovery.

The results? Despite the fact that over the 6 weeks the volunteers had done less than 10 minutes of hard exercise in total, they actually became fitter, showing significant improvements in the maximum amount of oxygen their body was able to utilize during exercise. Men had increased their volume by 15 percent and women by 12 percent.

Another study, co-authored by Martin Gibala, PhD, who has been in the forefront of HIIT, is also compelling. One group of students rode a bicycle for 1 to 2½ hours at a sustainable pace. Another group rode in intense 20- to 30-second bouts, after resting 4 minutes, and did so repeatedly four to six times more for a total of 6 minutes of exercise. Despite the vast difference in time expended, the two groups experienced the same benefit.[5] My point is not that you must do HIIT (although you may choose to do so as you advance in your exercise program), but that it's perfectly possible to benefit from short, intense periods of exercise.

When researchers had more than 4,500 volunteers wear accelerometers over a 3-year period to track the pace and duration of their physical activity, they found that repeated bursts of a mere 2 or 3 minutes of intense activity was as effective at preventing weight gain as 10 or more minutes of steady exercise.[6] Wait, it gets better. In another study, at the University of Western Ontario, where I got my undergraduate degree, men and women who did four to six 30-second sprints (after warming up) three times a week shed twice as much body fat over 6 weeks as a matched group of people who ran for 30 to 60 minutes three times a week.[7] The results gained in a fraction of time were equivalent to those achieved with hours of exercise. Again, short periods of intense exercise can yield impressive results.

In a study out of Japan, the subjects were rats, not humans, and the aerobic activity was swimming, not sprinting, but it also supports the value of interval training. The rats swam in tanks while wearing tiny vests—I kid you not—weighted to be equivalent to 14 to 16 percent of their body weight. One group swam for 6 hours a day and the other for a few minutes a day.[8] (Yes, you read that right.) The first group endured 3 hours of swimming, followed by a rest, and then 3 more hours back in the water. The other (lucky) rats swam for 20 seconds, had a 10-second rest, then another 20 seconds of swimming, and so forth, until they had exercised for about 4½ minutes. Despite the vast different in exercise time, the two groups experienced the *exact same* aerobic benefits.

STEP UP YOUR ACTIVITY

Climbing stairs is another great way to take things up a notch. No need to buy an expensive stair-climbing machine or join a health club. Unless you live in a house without stairs, you have an excellent way to enhance your aerobic fitness, right at your fingertips, or should I say tippy toes? The United States government has launched a national effort to counter the epidemic of

For Safety's Sake

Climbing stairs is great exercise, but take some precautions to avoid an accident or other incident.

- If you're not used to climbing lots of stairs, start with a slow pace and just one or two flights. Then pick up the pace and the number of flights.

- Walk for a few minutes first to warm up your muscles.

- Hold the handrail on the way down, but not up.

- Don't go up (or down) so fast that you're at risk of losing your balance.

- Going up puts hardly any stress on your joints; going down, however, does. If it hurts, simply go down sideways.

- Take a break if you feel dizzy or out of breath or if your thighs feel like they're burning up.

- Keep your back straight, lean forward slightly from the hips, and keep your eyes on the stairs.

- Place your entire foot on each step and drive with your heel.

- Only use stairs that are well lit.

- If you're in a public place, be sure you could call for help if you fell or felt threatened.

obesity with a program of 100 "small step" lifestyle changes, of which number 67 is using stairs instead of escalators in public places.[9]

Climbing stairs can also help extend your life. According to a long-running study of Harvard alumni, men who walk 1.3 miles a day have a 22 percent lower mortality rate than sedentary men. But men who climb an average of at least eight flights a day do even better: they have a 33 percent lower mortality rate than their sedentary peers.[10]

Climbing stairs combines both aerobic and resistance exercise as you both lift your body weight and increase your oxygen intake. Believe it or not, climbing stairs is more aerobically demanding than lifting a moderately heavy weight for an equivalent amount of time.[11] Climbing stairs also helps tone your buttocks, thighs, and legs and builds bone strength. And you'll burn two to three times as many calories as you would walking briskly on a level surface. So, if you're pressed for time, stair climbing can be an efficient form of activity. If you live in a high-rise apartment building, climbing stairs can be a great substitute for walking outdoors in inclement weather. Also check out shopping malls and multistory parking garages. Of course, going *down* stairs is not as taxing, but those steps also count toward your daily tally.

As you build your strength and endurance, extend the amount of time or number of steps. Also consider taking two steps at a time, which uses different and larger muscle groups, or wearing a weighted vest or backpack to increase resistance.

ON AN INCLINE

Assuming you're wearing the right shoes and walking on a flat surface, have you ever had the feeling that you could walk forever? It's an exhilarating experience. But when you're climbing a hill or walking on an inclined treadmill, you tend to slow down and breathe more heavily. By moving your body weight up the incline, you're increasing your dose of aerobic activity with some resistance exercise tossed in for good measure, just as you do when you climb stairs. No wonder you may feel a bit short of breath and start huffing and puffing. Like stair climbing, walking on an incline is a more efficient exercise because it burns more calories than walking on a level surface, with the added bonus of being easier on your joints while toning and defining your thigh, quads, glutes, and calf muscles. Bottom line: stronger legs and a firmer butt.

If you're a novice walker, once you're comfortable with a half-hour walk, find a place that combines flat and hilly surfaces so you can catch your breath between climbing hills. Or find a short and not-too-steep incline, perhaps in a shopping center parking lot, and walk up and down it a few times to get in practice. A treadmill may not offer the experience of being outdoors, but at least you can program it to alternate "hills" and flat surfaces, as well as control the incline of the "hills." A treadmill can also come in handy in inclement weather or when snow and ice make it dangerous to walk outdoors.

Six More Aerobic Activities to Explore

1. TAKE THE PLUNGE. Swimming is low impact, putting little stress on your joints, bones, and ligaments, so it's a good alternative if you have weak knees or other injuries.

2. TAKE A HIKE. Get out into the natural world and burn more calories than you would by simply walking on a city street or around your neighborhood. Hiking by yourself can be almost meditative, but going with a friend is safer and a great way to bond.

3. STRAP ON YOUR INLINE SKATES. And don't forget your kneepads and helmet. Your kids will love you for it!

4. DANCE TO YOUR OWN TUNE. In addition to getting a workout, you'll have fun and banish some stress. Take a Zumba or line-dancing class, or just turn on the radio and get your moves on.

5. PLAY BALL. Playing pickup basketball or doubles tennis is both fun and a great way to get an aerobic workout.

6. DO IT INDOORS. If you're pressed for time or facing adverse weather, heading to the gym to get your steps in on a cardio machine is a good option. I like the Cybex Arc Trainer, Helix Lateral Trainer, and Precor Elliptical.

THE NEXT LEVEL OF RESISTANCE EXERCISE

Resistance exercise is inherently simple to modify by increasing the number of sets and/or reps. These incremental increases are built into the Beginner, Intermediate, and Advanced level instructions you'll find starting on page 216. In exercises that call for the use of dumbbells rather than your own body weight, using a heavier weight obviously increases resistance. For the first 5 days on My 5, you've been doing about 5 minutes of resistance exercise daily, but increasing the number of minutes clearly ramps up the workout.

Boredom is the enemy of any activity. Just as I want you to explore more variety in your food choices, adding variety to your resistance exercises will make working out more interesting. Various exercises also work the same muscles in slightly different ways so your body continues to be challenged. (Once an exercise is too easy or done too frequently, its benefit decreases.) So for each of the seven major muscle groups, I've added an alternative exercise with which you can switch off. (Remember, it takes 7 days to include all muscle groups.) You can start doing these exercises after 6 weeks of doing the Basic exercises if you have reached the Advanced level. If not, continue until you do achieve that level. You'll find the alternate exercises in the Resistance Exercises section, starting on page 223 under the heading "Add Variety." And for those of you who want an even greater challenge once you've

Change It Up Some More

Other ways to add variety to your resistance exercise program include using different tools and different bases. For example, in addition to using your own body weight and dumbbells, you can experiment with resistance bands, kettle bells, cables, exercise balls, and exercise machines. Likewise, working the same muscle groups while lying down, sitting, kneeling, standing, using a bench, or lying on an exercise ball changes your base and therefore your experience. Check out these variations on Google or YouTube to see which appeal to you.

Advice for the Advanced

While you can train most of your body with minimal equipment to get in great shape, when you reach the advanced level, it can be beneficial to have access to a full gym a few times a month. That way you'll be able to train two body parts that are difficult to train at home effectively: lats (back) and adductors (inner thigh). A tiny percent of you may be able to do 15 to 20 pullups with ease on a bar installed in a doorway, but most of us simply cannot. Instead, you can benefit greatly from the efficiency (and safety) of a cable resistance machine.

reached the Advanced level of Add Variety, I've added more advanced resistance exercises to combine with some of those you are already doing. You'll find them starting on page 232 under "Take It Up a Notch."

Now let's get into more detail on each of these ways to up the ante:

- **ADVANCE TO THE NEXT LEVEL.** You'll recall that the Beginner, Intermediate, and Advanced exercises all involve three sets. The progression is in the number of repetitions per set, ranging from 10 to 20 to 30, respectively. If you've been at the Beginner level, after 4 weeks try moving up to Intermediate, doing 20 reps per set. Likewise, after another 4 weeks at the Intermediate level, move up to Advanced, doing 30 reps a set. If that is too great an increase, do what you can do, perhaps 15 or 25 reps, respectively, gradually building your strength.

- **INCREASE SETS, REPS, AND RESISTANCE.** By doing more sets and reps, you're obviously increasing the total amount of work done. In the case of the exercises that require dumbbells, you can also move to a heavier weight once you've become accustomed to doing more reps to further challenge yourself.

- **INTRODUCE VARIETY.** After the first 6 weeks on My 5, you can begin to swap exercises out with seven alternative ones that work the same muscle groups, assuming you have reached and spent at least 1 week at the Advanced level. You'll need an exercise ball to do one of these new exercises. Find photographs and instructions for the following exercises starting on page 224:

- Single-Leg Tap Squat instead of Reverse Lunge
- Hip Thrust instead of Superman
- Dumbbell Single-Arm Triceps Kickback instead of Lying Dumbbells Triceps Extension
- Ball Hamstring Curl instead of Stiff-Leg Dumbbell Deadlift
- Dumbbell Lateral Raise instead of Standing Dumbbell Curl Press
- Reverse Fly instead of Single-Arm Dumbbell Row
- Side Plank instead of Dumbbell Standing Side Bend

Five Key Points in Chapter 8

1. Continue to ask yourself the same five questions each day to ensure that you maintain your weight or continue to shed any remaining excess pounds. Answering each question with a yes remains an immediate and tangible way to measure your results.

2. Each day, continue to eat the same way, do your resistance exercises, walk at least 10,000 steps, sleep for at least 7 continuous hours, and unplug from electronics for at least 1 hour.

3. Add more variety to your meals with two "free" meals or snacks a week. Do more sets or reps of your resistance exercises, add more weight, and/or try some new moves. Gradually increase the number of daily steps you take. Begin to meditate or do yoga, perhaps in some of your unplugged time.

4. Weigh yourself once a month at the same time of day to get the most accurate gauge of your progress. People who weigh themselves regularly are more likely to keep banished pounds off for good.

5. As you get stronger, your body adapts, so you need to challenge it more. Add climbing stairs, walking on an incline, jogging, running, or interspersing short sprints with walking or running to your aerobic exercise program to burn more calories or burn them faster. Challenge yourself to move from the Beginner to Intermediate to Advanced resistance exercises when you're ready; and/or increase the weight of your dumbbells, and/or the number of reps; and/or try using resistance bands, an exercise ball, kettle ball, or other devices.

- **INCREASE THE NUMBER OF EXERCISES.** Once you're at the Advanced level and needing more of a challenge after a minimum of 6 weeks, add an incremental exercise to each session. This will increase your time from about 5 minutes to about 10. You'll be doing the following combo workouts, for which you'll find photographs and instructions starting on page 231.

  - Pike Plank and Reverse Lunge
  - Lying Dumbbell Triceps Extension and Hip Thrust
  - Standing Dumbbell Side Bends and Stiff-Leg Dumbbell Deadlift
  - Seated Trunk Twist and Standing Dumbbell Shoulder Press
  - Single-Arm Dumbbell Row and Superman
  - Dumbbell Hammer Biceps Curl and Plank
  - Sumo Squat or Pushup (for men only) and Lying Trunk Twist

Over the past 5 days, you've made some significant changes in your behavior. But doing anything for 5 days does not a habit make. In the next chapter, we'll talk about how to turn your new behaviors into habits that will become an integral part of your life so that you'll never regain those banished pounds and inches.

CHAPTER

9

WHY YOU'LL NEVER REGAIN THE POUNDS

We're all creatures of habit. To a large extent, that's a good thing. Habits allow us to handle the routine aspects of life without thinking about them. Long before *multitasking* became a buzzword, this ability allowed us to do two or more things at a time. If you don't have to think about doing something to make it happen, you can simultaneously give your attention to something else. That's why you can change a diaper, comfort your baby, and talk to your boss on the phone, all at the same time. Of course, a speakerphone helps too!

When you first learned to drive, you concentrated like crazy. There were so many things you had to be simultaneously aware of. But over time, driving becomes a habit. You find you can listen to your favorite radio station, all the while safely braking, parking, shifting gears, and doing all the other habitual moves associated with driving.

If you don't have to waste brainpower deciding whether to brush your teeth before washing your face or whether to have a cup of coffee before making breakfast for the family, it frees your mind up for other, more important or creative thoughts. President Obama made this point in an article in *Vanity Fair*. When writer Michael Lewis asked him to teach him how to be president, Obama first cited the importance of exercise and next the power of routine. "You'll see I wear only gray or blue suits," he said. "I'm trying to pare down decisions. I don't want to make decisions about what I'm eating or wearing. Because I have too many other decisions to make."[1]

GOOD (AND NOT SO GOOD) HABITS

You can be justly proud of your good habits, whether engaging your seatbelt as soon as you get in the car, picking up your housebound neighbor's mail when you get your own, or putting the dirty dishes in the dishwasher after every meal. Certain habits can also protect you and your loved ones: always checking that the stove is off before leaving the house, for example, or looking both ways before crossing the street. Habits become a form of cruise control. Then there are those habits you probably want to change. Whether it's eating in front of the TV, skipping breakfast, or watching TV for hours on end, they're the habits that produce results you're not happy with. We all have such habits—and we can all change them.

Full disclosure: I once had habits that are now history. I grew up visiting my Cuban cousins in Miami and got into the habit of drinking *café cortaditos*, which are full of sugar and condensed whole milk. Now I opt for low- or nonfat milk and give sugar a pass. Here's another habit that may surprise you: I used to skip cardio because I found zoning out on a treadmill boring. Today I make phone calls while I'm on the move and set up my meetings and social plans within walking distance. Growing up during the fat-free, "carbs are amazing" era, my regular late-night snack was Raisin Bran. Now I don't need to eat after dinner, and for a daytime snack equivalent, I'll opt for All-Bran or Kashi GoLean with some berries in Greek yogurt. And I used to put ketchup on everything, but now I've swapped it out for Tabasco or salsa.

I'm not telling you this to shock you with my former habits or impress you with my current ones, but to make a point. We can all change our habits, and replacing one habit with another habit is an effective strategy. It's far more productive than just feeling guilty and beating yourself up. Instead, acknowledging that you need to work on an unproductive habit is the first step to overcoming it. I won't deny that it takes work to change a habit, but you've already demonstrated that you have the potential to do so by your answers (and the actions upon which they were based) over the past 5 days.

BEHAVIOR AND HABIT: WHAT'S THE DIFFERENCE?

Our behavior is our response to our environment. Another person, a certain situation, or a new place triggers a certain response. You would probably react differently to a child asking for your help crossing a busy street in broad daylight than you might to a burly guy who tried to take your arm while you were traversing a deserted street at night. Behavior can be voluntary (being polite to strangers) or involuntary (losing your temper when you're frustrated by someone or something). Habits, on the other hand, are things you do subconsciously, almost automatically, without having to think about them. They're an acquired behavior pattern, something that you do so regularly it becomes almost involuntary. Habits help shape the routines of our life.

THE PATH TO NEW HABITS

Assuming that you're happy with the results you've achieved on My 5, you'll want to maintain or continue those results. After all, who doesn't want to feel slimmer and fitter, and more energetic, rested, and satiated. And yes, in control of your life!

This book is about changing your behavior for 5 days in order to lose 5 pounds. But the greater message is about a way of being that promotes good nutrition, fitness, good health, and a healthy weight, along with a sense of mastery and accomplishment. In the first 5 days, you practiced five results-oriented behaviors. I'm pretty sure that now you'll want these conscious behaviors to become ingrained habits because the reward is so, well, rewarding.

A study suggests that it can take as few as 18 days to form a habit.[2] Researchers at University College London had 96 students come up with a simple behavior related to food, fitness, or health to which they aspired. Over the next 84 days, each student logged onto a website to report on whether he or she had followed through on the new behavior and when it became automatic. The median time for the behavior to become a habit was 66 days. However, the easier it was to achieve the change, the fewer days on average it took for the behavior to become a habit. So drinking more water became a habit sooner than eating a piece of fruit with lunch, and doing 50 sets of a particular resistance exercise a day, for example, took longer. The overall range was from 18 to 254 days, depending on the individual and the habit, leading the researchers to conclude that a subgroup of people are more habit-resistant than others. Despite their stated goal, some students weren't able to turn a desired behavior into a habit.

MUSCLES, SELF-CONTROL, AND HABIT FORMATION

How much of the process of developing good habits is self-control? A provocatively titled study asked the question "Does self-control resemble a muscle?" After reviewing hundreds of earlier studies, the authors declared that it does.[3] Just as you can strengthen a muscle by exercising it regularly, you can strengthen your willpower over time and with repetition. The more you practice certain behaviors that you perceive as good for you, the stronger your commitment to sticking with that behavior. In other words, it becomes a habit.

Other researchers followed up on this meta-study, including two Australian scientists who wanted to see how willpower could be enhanced over time. In one study, they had a group of primarily sedentary people do resistance exercise and aerobic workouts three times a week. A control group made no changes in their lives. All the study subjects took a visual tracking test that measured willpower at the start, during, and at the end of the test period. The active group's results showed that exercise boosted their ability to resist tasks that sap willpower and to do well on activities that require willpower.[4] So exercise strengthened not just the subjects' bodies but also their willpower.

All well and good, but there's more. The study subjects also reported on a mixed bag of other aspects of their lives, including smoking, drinking alcohol, eating junk food, wasting money, losing their temper, doing homework, watching TV, and missing appointments. In each category, "bad" behavior declined dramatically and "good" behavior increased comparably among the active subjects. The process of exercising had spurred them to make numerous other positive changes in their lives. The control group, on the other hand, didn't see their habits change much. Our old friend synergy is at work again. In this case, establishing one new habit—exercise—triggered a ripple effect of other good habits. That's just what happens with My 5.

GOAL-ORIENTED

To form a habit, there must first be a goal, which distinguishes a habit from the mind's other automatic processes.[5] Not surprisingly, people are more likely to repeat behaviors that are rewarding or deliver a desired result. Some habits are stronger or weaker than others depending on the frequency with which they're practiced.[6] It takes a conscious decision—or mindfulness, if you prefer—to make the permanent changes in behavior that ultimately evolve into a strong habit. And just like you want to not only sleep for at least 7 hours a night but also to enjoy continuous quality sleep, you want to develop strong habits as well, not weak ones.

Losing 5 pounds on the My 5 program lays the groundwork for permanent behavioral changes that will allow you to reach your weight goal (if you have more than 5 pounds to lose) or end a pattern of yo-yo dieting (if you're now where you want to be). Now the challenge is to turn those positive behaviors into habits. How long it will take you to make your new behaviors habits depends on you, of course. You've consciously behaved a certain way for 5 days and you know how to evaluate those behaviors with a simple set of yes's or no's at the end of the day. So you have a definite leg up on the average person hoping to forge new habits. Plus, you're almost a week into the 66 days it takes for a behavior to become a habit, which of course is just an average. (You may well be one of those lucky people who can beat the average and develop new habits more quickly.) And also, unlike most people, you have a tangible way to know whether you're staying on track.

THE HABIT LOOP

Once you've completely internalized a behavior, whether it's letting the dog out as soon as you wake up or turning down the heat at night before going to bed, it becomes a habit. A trigger, such as waking up or heading for bed, cues your brain to go on autopilot and you shift mental gears into habit mode. Performing the habitual behavior provides a reward, which ensures its continuance. Letting the dog out means you won't have to clean up a puddle (or worse) and eliminates the need to get out of a comfy bed in the middle of the night when Fluffy starts whining. Turning down the thermostat saves you money.

You've undoubtedly heard the old saying "Old habits die hard." Part of the challenge of developing new habits is leaving behind some old habits—and they can exert a powerful pull on you. It's so much easier to fall back on old habits than it is to develop new ones. The former is subconscious; however, initially the desired replacement behavior is decidedly conscious. One way to change habits is to eliminate the trigger or mute its power. Take hunger, for example. Say that your trigger is feeling hungry after work. Your original habit was to skip lunch and pick up fast food on the way home. When you replace that habit with a new behavior—eating three meals and two snacks made up of foods that produce the "holy trinity" of satiety, namely protein, fibrous carbs, and healthy fats—you prevent activation of the trigger. Your rewards are many: You'll save money, lose weight, improve your health indicators, and feel empowered. Wow! All from saying good-bye to one habit and welcoming another.

TAME THOSE TRIGGERS

Of course, in your effort to banish unproductive habits, you must first identify the triggers. I used to go to a coffee shop that had the best cookies in the
world. I couldn't have a coffee without a gooey chocolate chip cookie. For a
while I fooled myself that I was there for the coffee, but then came to accept
the fact that I was really going there for the cookies. I now go to a different
coffee shop, one without the cookie trigger. If you've had a similar experience, you may even need to avoid the street where the tempting aromas spill
out of the shop. The same goes for certain snack foods and cereals you bring
into the house. If you have a hard time resisting them once they're in the
pantry, just say no—in the grocery aisle! Obviously, if you're determined to
stop smoking, you'll get rid of all the cigarettes in the house. If having the

Five Tips to Banish Bad Habits

1. ELIMINATE TEMPTATION. Don't bring anything into the house that
might serve as trigger.

2. TAKE A VACATION. In a radio interview, Charles Duhigg, author of *The
Power of Habit: Why We Do What We Do in Life and Business,* advised
that "changing a habit on a vacation is one of the proven most-successful
ways to do it . . . because all your old cues and all your old rewards aren't
there anymore. So you have this ability to form a new pattern and . . . carry
it over into your life."[7]

3. REPLACE A BAD HABIT WITH A GOOD HABIT. If watching television helps you unwind, replace it with meditating or reading to respond to
your need to relax.

4. ACCEPT THAT IT MAY NOT HAPPEN EASILY. Do your best, but
don't be discouraged if you experience a few bumps before you get there.
Just get up the next morning and focus on being able to answer yes five
times at the end of the day.

5. WRITE DOWN YOUR RESOLUTION. Declaring your intention on
paper (or on your computer) helps you focus on the end result. Continue to
answer the five questions in your journal and provide explanations if and
when your answer is no to help you spot any patterns.

Five Tips to Develop "Sticky" Habits

1. DO IT EVERY DAY. Consistency is key to establishing new habits.

2. USE REMINDERS. It's easy to get distracted by other matters, so don't rely on your memory alone. Use the alarm on your smartphone, entries in your Day-Timer, or good old-fashioned Post-it notes.

3. BE CONSISTENT. Doing is becoming. The more consistently you perform your new behavior, the easier it is to make it a habit. For example, do your resistance exercises in the same room at the same time every day. Such cues make it easier to stick to your resolutions.

4. FIND A BUDDY. Ask a friend or family member to join you on My 5. You'll both find it easier to stay motivated long-term.

5. CREATE A TRIGGER. If you have trouble with one of the five components of My 5, come up with a way to remind yourself. For example, set your alarm clock 15 minutes early (so long as it doesn't cut into your minimum of 7 hours of shut-eye) so that you can get out for a short walk first thing each day.

TV in the bedroom tempts you to watch shows late into the night, put it in another room. (That's a good idea in any case, as we discussed in Chapter 4.)

THE POWER OF REPETITION

Just as increasing the number of repetitions of each resistance exercise increases your strength and endurance, consistently repeating a certain behavior increases the likelihood it will become a habit. Remember, we can strengthen our willpower, just as we can strengthen our muscles, with regular "workouts." Following a personal schedule is a great way to establish the consistency necessary to ensure you do certain things at a certain time of day. It's 7:30 a.m.—time for my walk. It's 3 p.m.—time for my resistance exercises. It's 10 p.m.—time to turn off the TV and do my mindfulness meditation. Of course, eating your meals and snacks on a roughly 3-hour schedule is part of the process of habituation. The clock can be a valuable ally in forming good habits. Or set the timer on your smartphone or computer if you tend to get absorbed in your work and lose track of time.

MORE ON MINDFULNESS

I introduced the concept of mindfulness in Chapter 5. In addition to helping you wind down before bed or escape from the pressures of our electronically connected world, mindfulness can also play a role in turning behaviors into habits. All too often, we respond mindlessly to our thoughts by continuing the same patterns of behavior we've exhibited in the past. We want to change, but we feel powerless to effect that change. Eating too much of the wrong foods is a mindless response to the hunger thoughts that course through our brain. On the other hand, mindfulness promotes an awareness of what you're thinking, as well as an awareness that you don't necessarily have to act on it. (You needn't eat that Whopper just because your mind is sending hunger signals or because you're craving it.) Buddhists refer to this disconnect between thought and action as detachment.

Once you realize that you needn't act on an impulse (a thought), it helps you begin to break the cause-and-effect reaction between your thoughts or emotions and your actions. By consistently breaking this connection, the power of the trigger—in this case, hunger or craving—is weakened. (Eating every 3 hours or so also diminishes the hunger trigger.) Over time, practicing mindfulness helps you "rewire" your brain messaging, helping you to form new responses and new habits.

FREEDOM FROM (TOO MANY) CHOICES

Earlier, I mentioned the time-management seminar I took with Stephen Covey, who stressed that when you prioritize what's important rather than what's urgent, you can achieve great things. It aligns with the anecdote about President Obama saying he was paring down the colors of his suits to reduce

Psych Yourself Up

You know you need to make permanent changes in your habits and you've started the process with the program introduced in this book. But what if you're wavering or feeling guilty that you're not executing it perfectly in every category every day? Instead of beating yourself up, use these tools to get your head (and heart) in the right place.

- **MODIFY THE NEGATIVE.** When thoughts like "I can't do this" creep into your mind, finish the sentence with something like this: "But if I stick with it, it will get easier."

- **REMIND YOURSELF OF THE BENEFITS.** Review sections of this book that pertain to an area in which you may be having difficulty. If it's walking at least 10,000 steps a day, for example, take another look at the incredible benefits aerobic activity brings, including a longer life span. Note in your journal any changes you see in your energy level or mood on the days you answer yes to that question rather than no.

- **THINK ABOUT THE CONSEQUENCES.** Whether it's dreading bathing suit weather or not wanting to tempt fate as a member of a family with history of diabetes, remind yourself why you started this program in the first place.

Finally, stop worrying and start doing!

the number of decisions he had to make. Habits allow you to limit your choices, enabling you to focus on what's important in life. If these two individuals don't inspire you, there's solid research that comes to a similar conclusion. Too many choices can actually impair self-control and initiative.

In a series of seven experiments, scientists had subjects make decisions about choosing consumer products, college courses, or course materials.[8] A control group looked over the options but did not have to make choices. All the subjects were then asked to perform an unpleasant task such as drinking a nasty-tasting drink or holding their hands in ice water. The object was to see whether the stress of having to make choices (or not) among a large number of options interfered with their self-control and their ability to stay on task to achieve a goal. Those who had to make choices did significantly worse than those who didn't have to make choices.

Another one of the seven experiments involved subjects going to a shopping mall for a specific number of hours, reporting on how many decisions they had made, and then being asked to solve simple arithmetic problems. The more choices the shoppers had made, the worse their problem-solving skills. Another experiment looked at pleasurable decisions. When told to select items for a gift registry and later asked to solve math problems, results showed that the shorter the time subjects spent deciding on a gift, the less mentally draining it was. Regardless of whether making decisions is fun or drudgery, cognitive function is diminished with every choice made.

My point is this: Follow My 5 for 5 days and you'll achieve results. And the longer you practice these behaviors, the more you'll enjoy the rewards of losing weight and getting fit and the more time you'll have to focus on what really matters in your life. Instead of having to make choices each day about what to eat, whether to exercise, etc., you'll have internalized these behaviors into habits.

KEEP IT OFF

Sadly, the majority of people who lose weight regain it within a year. So what factors mark those who are successful in banishing those excess pounds for good? Maintaining the behaviors that led to weight loss is key, which is why extreme or "crash" diets don't work—they're impossible to maintain. The research on this subject is remarkably consistent. For example, in a study on the habits of individuals who'd lost and maintained an average weight loss of 37 pounds over 7 years, researchers found that in addition to following a weight-loss diet, they exercised regularly and weighed themselves regularly.[9] Two years after weight loss, when behavior patterns of "maintainers" were compared to "regainers" in another study, the former were more likely to continue the strategies they used while losing weight and to weigh in regularly. Not surprisingly, regainers, on the other hand, were less likely to continue the dietary and exercise strategies they had used while losing weight.[10]

Eating regular meals and specifically eating breakfast are also success markers. In a review of studies that looked at people who'd maintained their weight loss for at least 6 months, success was associated with greater initial weight loss; reaching a self-determined goal weight; being physically active; eating meals on a regular schedule, including breakfast; "healthier eating;" controlling overeating; and behavior self-monitoring.[11] Beginning to see a pattern?

A study that looked specifically at self-monitoring by women over a year-long weight-loss program found that individuals who weighed themselves regularly, kept a food journal, and monitored their energy intake were also less likely to engage in binge eating than individuals who did not.[12] Journaling, of course, is a traditional way to self-monitor. (See "Write It Down!" on page 244.) You'll find weight-monitoring programs online, and an array of weight-loss and weight-maintenance apps is also available.

The takeaway of all these studies is clear, and the findings are hardly surprising. Behaving one way for 5 days, 5 weeks, or 5 months—in other words, going on a "diet"—and then returning to the old way of eating is the all-too typical pattern. Not surprisingly, discouragement sets in when those lost pounds reappear, often along with a few more. The same can be said for a short-lived burst of enthusiasm for a new exercise machine or fitness program. To continue to lose weight or to maintain your new weight requires two basics: consistency of behavior and self-monitoring. My 5 behaviors provide the first; answering the five questions each day, the second. Which is why I'm asking you to continue to ask and answer the five questions daily and record the responses and any other comments in your journal.

There's a mouthful of a word, *eudemonic*, which refers to a sense of well-being, a purposeful engagement with life, a realization of your potential and ability to actualize it. Once you start to feel better about yourself, feel stronger, and feel a little slimmer, all those good things promote positive feelings. Feeling accomplished in one area of your life leads to greater confidence that you can achieve accomplishment in others. Now that you have achieved success on My 5, I'll bet that you'll be all fired up and empowered to make some other changes in your life. And I know you'll succeed.

Five Key Points in Chapter 9

1. Habits allow us to handle the routine aspects of life and focus instead on our conscious attention to other matters.

2. Behavior is a response to a specific environmental factor, while habits are things you do subconsciously, almost automatically, without having to think about them. A behavior can become a habit after it has been repeated regularly and consistently. Good habits can be strengthened, just as you strengthen a muscle with consistent workouts.

3. The three-part process known as a "habit loop" includes a trigger or cue, followed by the routine behavior, and then a reward, which reinforces the habit. To banish a habit, you have to interrupt that loop repeatedly until it breaks its hold on your brain.

4. Mindfulness can help turn behaviors into habits. Instead of responding mindlessly to our thoughts, mindfulness brings an awareness that you don't necessarily have to act on your thoughts and emotions, giving you greater self-control.

5. The My 5 Plan has already given you all the tools you need to form the habits that will keep you slim and trim. You just need to practice them daily and consistently.

And if you ever do regain weight, perhaps after having a baby or recuperating from an injury, rest assured that you now have the know-how and tools to get on the case immediately and banish 5 pounds in 5 days. Now turn the page to find all the resources you'll need to make My 5 as easy as possible: recipes; and instructions on how to do the resistance exercises, complete with photos; and journal pages to track your progress.

PART

3

RECIPES

RECIPE INDEX

SMOOTHIES

Green Ginger-Peach Smoothie 176

Blueberry-Pomegranate Slushie 177

Tropical Green Smoothie 178

PB and Grape Smoothie 179

Apple, Peach, and Spinach Smoothie 180

SCRAMBLES

Artichoke, Mushroom, and Smoked Salmon Scramble 181

Spinach Omelet with Feta and Avocado 182

South-of-the-Border Omelet 183

Sweet Potato Hash with Turkey Sausage 184

Italian Frittata with Zucchini, Leeks, and Parmesan 185

SANDWICHES

Salmon and Goat Cheese Melt 186

White Bean, Caramelized Onion, and Wilted Arugula Toast 187

Grilled Cheese, Pear, and Turkey Sandwich 188

Charred Corn and Cumin Chicken Wrap 189

SALADS

Curried Chicken and Baby Spinach Salad 190

Cumin-Roasted Sweet Potato, Quinoa,
and Black Bean Salad 191

Spicy, Crunchy Wheat Berry Salad 192

Kale Salad with Toasted Chickpeas
and Lemon-Tahini Dressing 193

Chopped Chicken and Pepperoni Salad on Mixed Greens 194

Salad Niçoise 196

SOUPS

Green Split Pea Soup 197

Manhattan-Style Chicken-Corn Chowder 198

Turkey, Barley, and Chard Soup 199

Mediterranean Lemon-Chicken Soup 200

Creamy White Bean and Kale Soup 201

STIR-FRIES AND SKILLET DISHES

Shrimp and Black Bean Stir-Fry 202

Saffron Shrimp Paella 203

Korean Chicken Stir-Fry 204

Spring Green Sauté with Farro 205

Steak and Ratatouille Stir-Fry 206

SNACKS

Lite French Toast 207

Bell Pepper and Turkey Roll-Ups 208

Red Lentil Puree 209

Pear Crumble with Greek Yogurt 210

Skinny Guacamole 211

Chocolate-Avocado Mousse with Raspberries 212

Berry-Muesli Yogurt Parfait 213

Note: Portion sizes assume a weight of up to 175 pounds. If you weigh more than that, increase portion sizes by one-third. Nutritional information reflects the regular serving size.

SMOOTHIES

GREEN GINGER-PEACH SMOOTHIE

Serves 1

Smoothies blend faster if you add the fruit and the liquid or yogurt at the same time. Add ice cubes to the mixture until the consistency is to your liking.

INGREDIENTS

1½ cups frozen peaches

¼ cup raspberries, fresh or frozen

1 teaspoon minced fresh ginger

½ cup nonfat plain Greek yogurt

1½ cups spinach leaves

6 whole raw almonds, coarsely chopped

1½ tablespoons (about ½ scoop) unflavored protein powder

Ice cubes (optional)

In a blender or food processor, blend the peaches, raspberries, ginger, yogurt, spinach, almonds, and protein powder until smooth. Add the ice cubes, if desired, and blend once more.

NUTRITION INFO: *315 calories, 25 grams protein, 37 grams carbs, 8 grams fiber, 9 grams fat*

BLUEBERRY-POMEGRANATE SLUSHIE

Serves 1

There are many types and brands of protein powder. My favorite is Source Organic Whey. Floating pomegranate seeds add texture and crunch to this frosty concoction.

INGREDIENTS

1 cup blueberries, fresh or frozen

¼ cup raspberries, fresh or frozen

½ cup nonfat milk

¼ cup pomegranate juice

1 tablespoon lime juice

3 tablespoons (about 1 scoop) unflavored protein powder

Ice cubes (optional)

2 tablespoons pomegranate seeds for garnish

In a blender or food processor, blend the blueberries, raspberries, milk, pomegranate juice, lime juice, and protein powder until smooth. Add the ice, if desired, and blend again. Garnish the drink with the pomegranate seeds.

NUTRITION INFO: *322 calories, 22 grams protein, 57 grams carbs, 8 grams fiber, 3 grams fat*

TROPICAL GREEN SMOOTHIE

Serves 1

Banana and avocado make a thick, fluffy drink. Add ice (or cold water) to thin it if you prefer.

INGREDIENTS

½ frozen banana, chopped

½ Hass avocado, peeled and chopped

½ cup mango slices, fresh or frozen

1 cup nonfat milk

1 tablespoon lime juice

1½ tablespoons (about ½ scoop) unflavored protein powder

Ice cubes (optional)

In a blender or food processor, blend the banana, avocado, mango, milk, lime juice, and protein powder until smooth. Add the ice cubes, if desired, and blend to the desired consistency.

NUTRITION INFO: *350 calories, 20 grams protein, 51 grams carbs, 8 grams fiber, 12 grams fat*

PB AND GRAPE SMOOTHIE

Serves 1

This riff on a peanut butter and jelly sandwich will make you feel like a kid again. Substitute skim milk for almond milk if you prefer, and/or almond butter for peanut butter. Follow the portion size guidelines on the protein powder container.

INGREDIENTS

½ cup unsweetened almond milk

½ small frozen banana, cut into chunks

½ cup green or red seedless grapes

1 cup chopped, cored, unpeeled apple

1 serving unsweetened protein powder

1½ teaspoons peanut butter

Ice cubes (optional)

In a blender or food processor, combine the almond milk, banana, grapes, apple, protein powder, and peanut butter. Add ice, if desired. Blend until the mixture reaches your desired consistency, thinning with a little water if necessary.

NUTRITION INFO: *336 calories, 28 grams protein, 45 grams carbs, 10 grams fiber, 6 grams fat*

APPLE, PEACH, AND SPINACH SMOOTHIE

Serves 1

Including a vegetable in your morning smoothie is a great way to boost your intake of fibrous carbs. If you like, swap kale, bok choy, or any other leafy green for the spinach; pineapple for the peach; and almonds for the macadamias.

INGREDIENTS

1 cup water (or more, depending on preferred texture)

1 cup chopped, cored, and unpeeled apple

3 cups chopped spinach

¾ teaspoon grated fresh ginger

1 medium peach, unpeeled and sliced

1 serving unsweetened protein powder

1 tablespoon macadamia nuts

Juice of 1 lemon (optional)

Ice cubes (optional)

Place the water, apple, spinach, ginger, peach, protein powder, nuts, and the lemon juice and ice cubes in a blender or food processor. Blend until the desired consistency is reached, adding more water to thin it out if necessary.

NUTRITION INFO: *290 calories, 27 grams protein, 44 grams carbs, 8 grams fiber, 5 grams fat*

SCRAMBLES

ARTICHOKE, MUSHROOM, AND SMOKED SALMON SCRAMBLE

Serves 2

To get this dish on the table ASAP, use pre-sliced mushrooms. Substitute two slices of high-fiber bread if you can't find the muffins.

INGREDIENTS

Cooking spray

2 tablespoons chopped onion

8 ounces button or baby bella mushrooms, sliced

12 frozen artichoke hearts

3 tablespoons water

8 egg whites (or 1 cup egg whites)

¼ cup skim milk

Salt and black pepper

3 tablespoons crumbled soft goat cheese

1 cup halved cherry tomatoes

3 ounces thinly sliced smoked salmon

2 high-fiber English muffins (Fiber One brand), halved and toasted

Fresh chives, chopped, for garnish (optional)

Heat a large nonstick sauté pan over medium-high heat. Coat with cooking spray. Add the onions and mushrooms; cook, stirring often, until they begin to soften, about 5 minutes. Stir in the artichokes and water. Cover the pan and cook for another 4 minutes, until the artichokes are cooked through and the water has evaporated.

Meanwhile, whisk together the egg whites and milk in a bowl. Season with salt and pepper. Add the egg mixture to the pan and gently cook, stirring constantly, until the eggs are completely cooked. Gently fold in the goat cheese, tomatoes, and salmon.

Top each half of an English muffin with the scramble. Garnish with chopped chives, if desired.

NUTRITION INFO: *362 calories, 40 grams protein, 42 grams carbs, 14 grams fiber, 9 grams fat*

SPINACH OMELET WITH FETA AND AVOCADO

Serves 2

Feta cheese is quite salty. Taste your omelet before seasoning it.

INGREDIENTS

Cooking spray

6 ounces baby spinach

¼ cup water

6 egg whites (or ¾ cup egg whites)

Salt and black pepper

4 tablespoons crumbled reduced-fat feta cheese

½ Hass avocado, peeled and sliced

2 high-fiber English muffins (Fiber One brand)

Lightly coat a medium nonstick skillet with cooking spray and place it over medium-low heat. Gradually add the spinach and the water. Cook for 4 minutes, until the water evaporates and the spinach is wilted, stirring occasionally. Transfer to a medium bowl.

In another medium bowl, whisk the egg whites, salt, and pepper.

Wipe the skillet with a paper towel and recoat it with cooking spray. Place it over medium heat and add the egg whites; cook for *3 seconds,* just until the edges start to set. Drawing the cooked egg to the center of the pan with a spatula, tilt the pan so the uncooked egg runs underneath the cooked part. Repeat all around the edge of the pan until the omelet is just set.

Drop the spinach mixture onto one half of the omelet and sprinkle with the feta. Cook for *10 to 20 seconds.* Run the spatula around the omelet to loosen the edges. Jerk the pan sharply to move the entire omelet. Tilt the pan, resting the edge on a serving plate. Gently roll the omelet onto the plate, using the spatula to fold it over the filling. Garnish with the avocado slices and serve with toasted muffins.

NUTRITION INFO: *278 calories, 22 grams protein, 39 grams carbs, 16 grams fiber, 9 grams fat*

SOUTH-OF-THE-BORDER OMELET

Serves 2

Egg whites cook more quickly than whole eggs, but once you learn the technique, you can have breakfast on the table in a flash. Fresh salsa usually has no added sugar, but check the label on jarred salsa.

INGREDIENTS

1 Hass avocado, peeled and diced

¾ cup canned black beans, drained and rinsed

¼ cup prepared salsa

1 teaspoon olive oil

1 whole egg

4 egg whites (or ½ cup egg whites)

Salt and black pepper

¼ cup shredded low-fat cheddar cheese

2 tablespoons chopped fresh cilantro

In a medium bowl, combine the avocado, beans, and salsa.

Warm the oil in a medium nonstick skillet over medium-high heat. In a medium bowl, beat the egg, egg whites, salt, and pepper. Once the pan is hot, add the egg mixture. Let the egg sit for 3 seconds, until the edges begin to set. Using a spatula, draw the lightly cooked egg to the center of the pan. Tilt the pan to the side so that the uncooked egg runs to the bare spot at the edge of the pan. Repeat the process all around the edge of the pan until the omelet is just set but still moist in the center.

Gently place the avocado filling evenly over half of the omelet. Sprinkle the filling with the cheese and cilantro. Cook for 20 seconds. Run the spatula quickly along the side of the omelet to loosen the edges. Jerk the pan sharply away from you a few times; the omelet should slide up the far side of the pan. Tilt the pan, resting the edge on a serving plate. Gently roll the omelet onto the plate, using the spatula to fold it over the filling.

NUTRITION INFO: *320 calories, 26 grams protein, 23 grams carbs, 8 grams fiber, 12 grams fat*

SWEET POTATO HASH WITH TURKEY SAUSAGE

Serves 2

When using only a small amount of oil in cooking, as in this hearty hash, keep an eagle eye on the skillet to make sure the sausage and vegetables don't burn.

INGREDIENTS

1 medium sweet potato, peeled and diced

3 ounces turkey sausage, crumbled

1 teaspoon olive oil

1 small onion, thinly sliced

1 clove garlic, minced

¼ teaspoon paprika

Salt and black pepper

4 egg whites (or ½ cup egg whites)

2 tablespoons minced fresh parsley for garnish

Preheat the oven to 400°F. Place the diced potatoes in a shallow microwave-safe bowl with enough water to barely cover them. Cover with plastic wrap and microwave for 2 minutes, until just tender. Drain.

In a medium cast-iron or heavy skillet over medium heat, cook the sausage for 5 minutes, until browned and starting to crisp, stirring often. Push the sausage to the edges of the pan. Reduce the heat to medium-low; add the oil, onion, garlic, and potatoes. Season with paprika, salt, and pepper. Cook for 8 minutes, until crisp and cooked through, stirring often.

Using the back of a serving spoon, make four wells in the mixture; evenly pour the egg whites into the wells.

Transfer to the oven; bake for 6 minutes, until the potatoes are hot and the eggs are baked through. Adjust the seasonings if necessary, and garnish with the parsley.

NUTRITION INFO: *342 calories, 19 grams protein, 53 grams carbs, 8 grams fiber, 6 grams fat*

ITALIAN FRITTATA WITH ZUCCHINI, LEEKS, AND PARMESAN

Serves 2

Leeks are often full of the soil in which they were grown, making them a pain to clean. Frozen leeks are great alternative without any loss of flavor. Or substitute two bunches of scallions.

INGREDIENTS

Cooking spray

2 leeks, thinly sliced and rinsed clean (white and pale green parts only)

1 small zucchini, diced

Salt and black pepper

2 whole eggs

3 egg whites (or ½ cup egg whites)

½ cup chopped fresh basil

⅓ cup grated reduced-fat Parmesan or Asiago cheese

4 slices high-fiber bread (Nature's Own, Mestermacher, or Food for Life Ezekiel 4:9), toasted

Preheat the oven to 350°F. Lightly coat a medium ovenproof nonstick skillet with cooking spray and place it over medium heat. Add the leeks and zucchini and season with salt and pepper. Cook for 5 minutes, until softened, stirring occasionally. Transfer the vegetables to a bowl.

In another bowl, beat the eggs and egg whites until well blended.

Using a paper towel, wipe out the skillet. Lightly coat it again with cooking spray and place it over medium heat. Add the eggs and egg whites and top them with the cooked leek-zucchini mixture, basil, and cheese. Cook for 2 minutes without stirring.

Transfer to the oven and bake for 8 to 10 minutes, until just set. Cut into wedges and serve directly out of the skillet while warm, accompanied by toast.

NUTRITION INFO: *366 calories, 24 grams protein, 50 grams carbs, 9 grams fiber, 11 grams fat*

SANDWICHES

SALMON AND GOAT CHEESE MELT

Serves 2

A single pita or a slice of high-fiber bread should contain at least 4 grams of fiber and 3 grams of protein and no more than 100 calories. In place of canned salmon, you can use vacuum-packed salmon, which doesn't need to be drained and patted dry.

INGREDIENTS

1 can (6 ounces) salmon packed in water, drained and patted dry

2 teaspoons olive oil

1 teaspoon red wine vinegar

Salt and black pepper

1 large tomato, cored and thinly sliced (about 6 slices)

1 ounce soft goat cheese, crumbled

1 teaspoon chopped fresh oregano or ½ teaspoon dried

3 high-fiber pitas, cut into wedges, or 3 slices high-fiber bread, toasted and cut into triangles

In a small bowl, toss the salmon, oil, and vinegar. Add salt and pepper to taste. Set aside.

Arrange the tomato slices, overlapping them slightly, on a large microwave-safe plate. Top with the salmon mixture and the goat cheese. Microwave or put the plate in a toaster oven for 2 minutes, until the cheese bubbles and the salmon is warmed through. Sprinkle with the oregano.

Serve hot with the pita wedges or bread.

NUTRITION INFO: *330 calories, 32 grams protein, 24 grams carbs, 9 grams fiber, 12 grams fat*

WHITE BEAN, CARAMELIZED ONION, AND WILTED ARUGULA TOAST

Serves 2

Caramelizing onions brings out their sweetness. Give them time to cook over a low flame until they become golden and melted.

INGREDIENTS

1 teaspoon olive oil

1 small yellow onion, thinly sliced

1 teaspoon chopped fresh thyme or ¼ teaspoon dried

Salt and black pepper

1 cup plus 2 tablespoons canned white kidney or cannellini beans, drained and rinsed

1½ cups (about 2 ounces) baby arugula

2 high-fiber pitas

Warm the oil in a medium nonstick skillet over medium-low heat. Add the onion and cook for 5 minutes, stirring occasionally. Reduce the heat to very low, cover the pot, and cook for 10 minutes, stirring often, until the onions are golden. Season with the thyme, salt, and pepper.

Increase the heat to medium, and stir in the beans and the arugula. Cook for 1 minute, until the beans are warmed through and the arugula wilts, stirring occasionally. If needed, add a tablespoon of water so the mixture doesn't stick to the pan.

Meanwhile, preheat a toaster oven to 300°F. Warm the pitas for 5 minutes, or until they're lightly toasted.

To serve, scoop the white bean mixture into the warm pitas.

NUTRITION INFO: *340 calories, 24 grams protein, 35 grams carbs, 8 grams fiber, 6 grams fat*

GRILLED CHEESE, PEAR, AND TURKEY SANDWICH

Serves 1

This childhood favorite gets a healthy makeover and tastes better than ever!

INGREDIENTS

1 teaspoon olive oil

2 slices high-fiber bread

½ ounce Swiss cheese, thinly sliced

½ small pear, thinly sliced

1 ounce turkey, thinly sliced

Several baby spinach leaves

Warm the oil in a small nonstick skillet over low heat. Layer a slice of bread with the cheese, pear, turkey, and spinach. Top with the remaining slice of bread.

Set the sandwich in the heated skillet. Set another heavy skillet on top of the sandwich to weight it down. Cook it for 2 minutes, until golden brown. Remove the weighting skillet and flip the sandwich. Replace the skillet and cook for 2 minutes, until the second side is golden brown.

Slice and serve warm.

NUTRITION INFO: *348 calories, 21 grams protein, 54 grams carbs, 12 grams fiber, 9 grams fat*

CHARRED CORN AND
CUMIN CHICKEN WRAP

Serves 1

In summer, use corn sliced off the cob and garden-fresh tomatoes. Off-season, frozen corn and cherry tomatoes make fine substitutes.

INGREDIENTS

½ cup corn kernels

1 tablespoon minced red onion

½ teaspoon ground cumin

1¾ ounces cooked chicken breast, shredded (about ¼ cup)

¼ cup chopped cherry or beefsteak tomatoes

2 tablespoons minced red bell pepper

2 teaspoons lime juice

Salt and black pepper

1 high-fiber tortilla, warmed

Warm a small nonstick skillet over medium-low heat. Add the corn, onion, and cumin, and toast for 2 minutes, until the corn becomes slightly charred, stirring often.

Remove the skillet from the heat; stir in the chicken, tomatoes, bell pepper, lime juice, salt, and pepper.

Mound the mixture on the warmed tortilla, wrap, and serve.

NUTRITION INFO: *350 calories, 29 grams protein, 44 grams carbs, 9 grams fiber, 9 grams fat*

SALADS

CURRIED CHICKEN AND BABY SPINACH SALAD

Serves 2

An array of flavors, textures, and colors makes this salad as pretty as it is tasty. Swap out other herbs, nuts, or fruits to suit your taste or use what's in your fridge. For a speedy no-cook dinner, pick up a rotisserie chicken, discard the skin, and shred the breast meat.

INGREDIENTS

1 container (4 ounces) plain nonfat Greek yogurt

1 tablespoon lime juice

1 teaspoon curry powder

4 ounces cooked chicken breast, shredded

1 stalk celery, thinly sliced

1 scallion, thinly sliced

Salt and black pepper

½ cup fresh raspberries

3 cups baby spinach

2 tablespoons chopped fresh cilantro

18 whole raw almonds, coarsely chopped

2 slices high-fiber bread, toasted and cut into triangles

In a medium bowl, whisk the yogurt, lime juice, and curry powder. Fold in the shredded chicken, celery, and scallion. Season to taste with salt and pepper. Gently fold in the raspberries.

Divide the spinach between two shallow serving bowls. Add a scoop of chicken salad to each plate; garnish with cilantro and almonds.

Serve with toast triangles for scooping.

NUTRITION INFO: *305 calories, 30 grams protein, 22 grams carbs, 10 grams fiber, 7 grams fat*

CUMIN-ROASTED SWEET POTATO, QUINOA, AND BLACK BEAN SALAD

Serves 2

The delicate texture of quinoa is a perfect partner to hearty sweet potatoes and black beans, but you can also substitute farro. Serve warm or at room temperature.

INGREDIENTS

1 small sweet potato, peeled and cut into 1-inch cubes

1 teaspoon olive oil

½ teaspoon ground cumin

Salt and black pepper

½ cup quinoa

1 cup water

3 tablespoons lime juice

1 cup canned black beans, drained and rinsed

1 tablespoon minced red onion

¼ cup chopped fresh cilantro

1 cup baby arugula

2 tablespoons crumbled, reduced-fat feta cheese

Preheat the oven to 400°F. On a baking sheet, toss the sweet potato cubes with the oil, cumin, salt, and pepper. Roast for 25 minutes, stirring occasionally, until the potatoes are tender on the inside and slightly crispy on the outside.

Meanwhile, in a small saucepan over high heat, bring the quinoa and water to a boil. Reduce the heat to low, cover, and simmer for 18 minutes, until the water is absorbed and the quinoa is fluffy. Remove the pan from the heat and let it sit, covered, for 5 minutes. Fluff the quinoa with a fork. If serving the salad at room temperature, refrigerate it for at least 15 minutes.

In a serving bowl, toss the sweet potatoes and quinoa with the lime juice, beans, onion, and cilantro. Line two serving plates with arugula, mound the quinoa mixture on top, and sprinkle with the feta.

NUTRITION INFO: *355 calories, 17 grams protein, 60 grams carbs, 12 grams fiber, 6 grams fat*

SPICY, CRUNCHY WHEAT BERRY SALAD

Serves 2

Available in specialty food stores and large supermarkets, wheat berries are the whole grain from which wheat flour is milled. They're a flavorful, fiber-rich substitute for rice or pasta. If you can't find wheat berries, use brown rice or quinoa. Serve warm, cold, or at room temperature.

INGREDIENTS

2/3 cup wheat berries

Pinch of salt

2 tablespoons lemon juice

1/2 teaspoon ground cinnamon

1 tablespoon minced red onion

1 small stalk celery, thinly sliced

3 tablespoons chopped walnuts

1/2 large crisp apple, diced

2 cups baby spinach

4 tablespoons soft goat cheese

In a small saucepan, combine the wheat berries and salt with water to cover by at least 2 inches. Place the pan over high heat and bring to a boil. Reduce the heat and simmer for 40 minutes, until the wheat berries are just tender but still have some bite.

Drain the wheat berries and toss them with the lemon juice and cinnamon. Let them cool slightly.

In a medium serving bowl, combine the onion, celery, walnuts, and apple. Fold in the cooled wheat berries.

Just before serving, divide the spinach between two serving plates. Mound the wheat berry mixture on top of the spinach. Top with the goat cheese.

NUTRITION INFO: *340 calories, 19 grams protein, 24 grams carbs, 10 grams fiber, 10 grams fat*

KALE SALAD WITH TOASTED CHICKPEAS AND LEMON-TAHINI DRESSING

Serves 1

Kale is a super-healthy alternative to lettuce. The tahini dressing, made with ground sesame seeds, tastes great on just about anything. Double the batch and use it another day drizzled over roasted vegetables.

INGREDIENTS

¾ cup canned chickpeas, drained and rinsed

Salt and black pepper

Pinch of ground cumin

1 tablespoon lemon juice

1 teaspoon tahini

1 small clove garlic, minced

2½ cups stemmed and chopped fresh kale leaves (about ½ bunch)

½ cup shredded carrot

Preheat the oven to 400°F.

On a rimmed baking sheet, toss the chickpeas with the salt, pepper, and cumin. Roast for 15 to 20 minutes, until crisp and lightly toasted, shaking the pan occasionally to ensure even toasting.

Meanwhile, in a medium serving bowl, whisk the lemon juice, tahini, and garlic until combined. Whisk in about 2 tablespoons water until the dressing is smooth and of the desired consistency.

Add the kale, carrot, and chickpeas; toss to coat well. Add more salt and pepper to taste.

NUTRITION INFO: *350 calories, 18 grams protein, 66 grams carbs, 13 grams fiber, 6 grams fat*

CHOPPED CHICKEN AND PEPPERONI SALAD ON MIXED GREENS

Serves 2

Turkey pepperoni, made by Hormel and other brands, is less fatty than but just as flavorful as salami.

INGREDIENTS

VINAIGRETTE

1 tablespoon chopped fresh basil or 1 teaspoon dried

1 tablespoon grated reduced-fat Parmesan cheese

2 tablespoons red wine vinegar

2 teaspoons olive oil

1 teaspoon Dijon mustard

SALAD

5 cups finely chopped romaine lettuce

2 cups finely chopped fresh spinach

4 ounces cooked skinless chicken breast, chopped

1 ounce sliced low-fat turkey pepperoni, chopped

1 medium English cucumber, unpeeled and chopped (about 2 cups)

5 fresh basil leaves, chopped

2 cups halved or quartered cherry tomatoes

½ cup canned chickpeas, drained and rinsed

2 tablespoons crumbled, reduced-fat feta cheese

Salt and black pepper

4 black olives for garnish

For the vinaigrette: In a small bowl, combine the basil, Parmesan, vinegar, oil, and mustard. Whisk until well blended. Set aside.

For the salad: In a large bowl, toss together the romaine and spinach. Divide between two plates.

In the same large bowl, combine the chicken, pepperoni, cucumber, basil, tomatoes, chickpeas, and feta; toss well. Spoon the mixture over the salad greens. Season with salt and pepper to taste.

Dress the salad with vinaigrette right before serving and garnish each plate with 2 olives.

NUTRITION INFO: *330 calories, 32 grams protein, 24 grams carbs, 9 grams fiber, 12 grams fat*

SALAD NIÇOISE

Serves 2

You can substitute canned shrimp or salmon for the tuna. You can also find both tuna and salmon in vacuum-pack bags. Wasa, Finn Crisp, RyKrisp, and Ryvita all make high-fiber crispbread.

INGREDIENTS

4 ounces green beans, trimmed and cut in half

1 can (6 ounces) light tuna packed in water, drained and patted dry

4 tablespoons red wine vinegar, divided

Salt

4 cups baby lettuce

1 medium tomato, cored and thinly sliced

1 tablespoon olive oil

2 hard-boiled eggs, yolks discarded

4 slices high-fiber Scandinavian crispbread

Bring a small saucepan of water to a boil over high heat. Add the beans and cook them for 3 minutes, until crisp-tender. Drain and rinse them with cool water.

In a small bowl, mix the tuna and 2 tablespoons of the vinegar. Season to taste with salt.

Arrange the lettuce, tomato slices, beans, and tuna evenly on two plates. Drizzle with the olive oil and the remaining 2 tablespoons vinegar. Slice the egg whites and arrange half on each plate, along with 2 slices of crispbread.

NUTRITION INFO: *356 calories, 31 grams protein, 42 grams carbs, 12 grams fiber, 9 grams fat*

GREEN SPLIT PEA SOUP

Serves 4

You can substitute yellow split peas for green ones. The soup will be just as tasty but will be a golden yellow color. If you have an immersion blender, skip Step 3 and puree the soup in the pot.

INGREDIENTS

½ teaspoon olive oil

6 ounces turkey bacon, chopped

2 medium carrots, chopped

1 small onion, chopped

1 stalk celery, chopped

Salt and black pepper

1¼ cups green split peas, washed and picked over

1 teaspoon fresh mint or ½ teaspoon dried

4 cups reduced-sodium chicken or vegetable broth

2 slices high-fiber bread, toasted and cut into triangles

Warm the oil in a medium saucepan over medium-low heat. Add the turkey bacon, carrots, onion, and celery; season with salt and pepper. Cook for 5 minutes, stirring often.

Add the split peas, mint, and broth. Bring to a boil; reduce the heat to a simmer and cook for 40 minutes, stirring often and adding up to 1 cup of water to maintain a soupy consistency.

Using a mug or ladle, remove about half of the soup. Puree it in a blender and return it to the pot. Warm it through, adding more broth if the soup seems too thick. Adjust the seasonings if necessary.

Serve with the toast triangles.

NUTRITION INFO: *390 calories, 28 grams protein, 51 grams carbs, 7 grams fiber, 7 grams fat*

MANHATTAN-STYLE CHICKEN-CORN CHOWDER

Serves 4

Depending on the season and your locale, fresh clams can be hard to come by, so chicken makes a great replacement in this satisfying chowder. You can also use chunks of salmon fillet.

INGREDIENTS

Cooking spray

2 slices turkey bacon, diced (optional)

4 cups diced unpeeled potatoes (any kind)

1 cup chopped onion

1 cup diced red bell pepper

2 tablespoons tomato paste

1¼ cups canned diced tomatoes

4 cups reduced-sodium chicken broth

9 ounces skinless chicken breast, cut into bite-size pieces

1½ cups corn kernels, frozen or canned

2 tablespoons chopped fresh tarragon or 2 teaspoons dried

Salt and black pepper

Heat a soup pot over medium heat. Mist it with cooking spray. Add the bacon, if using, and cook until crisp. Remove and set aside.

Add the potatoes, onions, and bell pepper. Cook, stirring often, until they begin to brown, about 6 minutes. Add the tomato paste and stir to coat the vegetables. Stir in the diced tomatoes, including the juice, and the broth. Bring to a boil.

Stir in the chicken, corn, and tarragon. Reduce the heat and simmer, uncovered, until the broth has thickened and the chicken is cooked through, about 20 minutes.

Season to taste with salt and pepper. Ladle into four bowls and garnish with the bacon, if desired.

NUTRITION INFO: *360 calories, 27 grams protein, 51 grams carbs, 7 grams fiber, 7 grams fat*

TURKEY, BARLEY, AND CHARD SOUP

Serves 4

This soup is extremely versatile. Instead of chard, use spinach or kale. Or use leftover cooked chicken or turkey and/or leftover cooked vegetables. To really speed things up, substitute leftover brown rice or quinoa for the pearl barley and eliminate the final simmering.

INGREDIENTS

2 teaspoons olive oil

1 cup chopped onion

8 ounces turkey breast, diced

Salt and black pepper

2 cups chopped carrots

1 cup chopped celery

4 cups chopped Swiss chard

6 cups reduced-sodium chicken broth

¾ cup pearl barley

1 tablespoon chopped fresh parsley or 1 teaspoon dried

1 tablespoon chopped fresh thyme or 1 teaspoon dried

Place a soup pot over medium-high heat; add the oil and heat. Add the onion and turkey and season with salt and pepper. Sauté, stirring occasionally, until the turkey is cooked through, about 7 minutes. Add the carrots and celery and sauté until soft. Stir in the chard and cook until it wilts.

Add the chicken broth and bring to a boil. Stir in the barley, parsley, and thyme.

Reduce the heat to low, cover, and simmer until the barley is tender, at least 45 minutes, adding water, if necessary.

Ladle into four bowls and serve.

NUTRITION INFO: *392 calories, 29 grams protein, 57 grams carbs, 12 grams fiber, 8 grams fat*

MEDITERRANEAN LEMON-CHICKEN SOUP

Serves 2

Leeks, lemon, dill, and spinach star in this vibrant chicken soup. Although it may seem like a lot of spinach, it cooks down. Use a rotisserie chicken or cooked, shredded chicken from the deli section. Use frozen leeks if you prefer.

INGREDIENTS

2 teaspoons olive oil

1 small leek, very thinly sliced and rinsed clean

½ stalk celery, thinly sliced

1 clove garlic, minced

1 teaspoon minced lemon zest

1 can (13¾ ounces) reduced-sodium chicken broth

½ cup shredded white-meat chicken

1 cup canned chickpeas, drained and rinsed

3 cups baby spinach

1 tablespoon lemon juice

1 tablespoon chopped fresh dill

Warm the oil in a medium saucepan over medium-low heat. Add the leek and celery and cook for 4 minutes, stirring occasionally. Add the garlic and lemon zest and cook for 1 minute, stirring occasionally. Add the broth and bring to a boil over high heat. Cook for 2 minutes.

Reduce the heat to medium. Stir in the chicken and chickpeas and cook for 2 minutes, until warmed through. Just before serving, stir in the spinach and lemon juice. Top each serving with dill.

NUTRITION INFO: *325 calories, 26 grams protein, 36 grams carbs, 8 grams fiber, 9 grams fat*

CREAMY WHITE BEAN AND KALE SOUP

Serves 2

I call this a pantry soup. If you have frozen chopped kale in the freezer, you just might already have everything on hand you need to make it. More good news: It can be ready in about 20 minutes! For a thicker soup, use a wooden spoon to mash some of the beans against the side of the pot while cooking.

INGREDIENTS

2 teaspoons olive oil

½ small onion, diced

2 large cloves garlic, minced

½ cup canned diced tomatoes, with juice

1 cup stemmed and chopped kale leaves

Salt and black pepper

1 can (13¾ ounces) reduced-sodium chicken broth

½ cup water

1 can (15 ounces) white beans, drained and rinsed

2 tablespoons finely grated Parmesan cheese

Warm the oil in a medium saucepan over medium-low heat. Add the onion and garlic and cook for 3 minutes, stirring often, until softened. Stir in the tomatoes and their juices and cook for 2 minutes.

Add the kale, season with salt and pepper, and cook for 3 minutes, stirring often, until the kale wilts.

Pour in the broth and the water, raise the heat, and bring it to a simmer. Add the beans. Simmer for 15 minutes, stirring occasionally and adding more water if needed.

Ladle into two bowls and garnish with the cheese.

NUTRITION INFO: *317 calories, 21 grams protein, 42 grams carbs, 10 grams fiber, 8 grams fat*

SHRIMP AND BLACK BEAN STIR-FRY

Serves 2

You can use frozen or canned shrimp. To save time, precooked brown rice is sold frozen at health food stores. Or make brown rice or quinoa ahead of time and freeze in meal-size portions.

INGREDIENTS

1 teaspoon sesame oil, divided

½ small onion, chopped

1 egg white, lightly beaten

1 teaspoon peeled and minced fresh ginger or ½ teaspoon ground

1 small jalapeño chile pepper, seeded and chopped

4 ounces frozen precooked (peeled and deveined) small shrimp, thawed

1½ cups cooked brown rice (or quinoa)

¼ cup canned black beans, drained and rinsed

2 tablespoons lemon juice

Place ½ teaspoon of the sesame oil in a large skillet over medium heat. Add the onion and cook for 3 minutes, until softened. Add the egg white, and cook for 1 minute without stirring. Using a wooden spoon, fold the egg white over so that it cooks through. Scrape the egg-onion mixture onto a platter.

Coat the pan again with the remaining ½ teaspoon of sesame oil and set it over medium heat. Stir in the ginger and jalapeño and cook for 30 seconds, stirring occasionally. Add the shrimp and cook for 2 minutes. Stir in the rice, beans, and egg mixture and cook until it's warmed through.

Divide between two serving plates. Drizzle with the lemon juice.

NUTRITION INFO: *280 calories, 18 grams protein, 43 grams carbs, 5 grams fiber, 4 grams fat*

SAFFRON SHRIMP PAELLA

Serves 2

Saffron lends a bright yellow hue as well as a subtle taste to any dish. If you don't have any around, ½ teaspoon of turmeric will add color. In lieu of quinoa, you can use cooked brown rice—just reduce the cooking time to 5 minutes.

INGREDIENTS

1 tablespoon olive oil

1 small onion, chopped

½ red bell pepper, seeded and chopped

3 cloves garlic, chopped

¼ teaspoon saffron threads, crumbled

¼ teaspoon hot paprika

Salt and black pepper

1 can (14½ ounces) reduced-sodium chicken broth

½ cup quinoa

6 ounces frozen precooked (peeled and deveined) large shrimp, thawed

½ cup frozen small peas, thawed

In a medium heavy skillet with 2-inch-high sides, warm the oil over medium heat. Add the onion and bell pepper and cook for 6 minutes, stirring often, until softened.

Stir in the garlic, saffron, paprika, and salt and pepper. Add the broth and quinoa. Bring to a boil. Reduce the heat to low, cover, and simmer for 12 minutes, until the quinoa is almost tender. Nestle the shrimp and peas in the quinoa, and add ¼ cup (or more) water to moisten, if necessary. Cover and cook until the shrimp are just opaque in the center, about 5 minutes. Adjust seasonings, if necessary, before serving.

NUTRITION INFO: *368 calories, 25 grams protein, 42 grams carbs, 6 grams fiber, 12 grams fat*

KOREAN CHICKEN STIR-FRY

Serves 2

You can have this complete meal on the table in a trice. Both udon and cellophane noodles cook quickly. Look for them in the Asian products section of your supermarket. You'll find precooked chicken breast in the deli section, or use leftover chicken. Or substitute leftover beef or pork.

INGREDIENTS

3 ounces cellophane or udon noodles

2 teaspoons olive oil

1 small onion, thinly sliced

3 cloves garlic, finely chopped

4 ounces fresh baby spinach (or 1 package frozen chopped spinach)

3 scallions, chopped

3 shiitake mushrooms, stemmed, wiped clean, and sliced

4 ounces cooked chicken breast, shredded

2 tablespoons reduced-sodium soy sauce

1 teaspoon dark sesame oil

Cook the noodles according to the package directions. Drain and rinse under cold water to prevent them from sticking.

Meanwhile, place a large skillet or wok over medium-high heat and add the olive oil. When the oil shimmers, add the onion and garlic and cook for 2 minutes, stirring often. Add the spinach, scallions, and mushrooms and cook for 4 minutes. Do not overcook. The vegetables should remain crispy.

Reduce the heat to low. Add the chicken, cooked noodles, soy sauce, and sesame oil. Cook for 2 minutes, tossing to combine the flavors and warm through before serving.

NUTRITION INFO: *374 calories, 22 grams protein, 51 grams carbs, 5 grams fiber, 9 grams fat*

SPRING GREEN SAUTÉ WITH FARRO

Serves 2

Farro is a fiber-rich ancient grain with a mild, nutty flavor. If unavailable, substitute barley, quinoa, or brown rice. Stir-frying asparagus and peas in a skillet rather than steaming them imparts a nice toasty flavor.

INGREDIENTS

¾ cup farro

3 cups water

1 teaspoon olive oil

4 ounces thin asparagus spears, sliced on the diagonal into ½-inch pieces

1 cup green peas, fresh or frozen

1 scallion, thinly sliced (white and pale green parts only)

4 tablespoons chopped fresh parsley

2 teaspoons lemon zest

2 tablespoons lemon juice

Salt and black pepper

½ cup part-skim ricotta cheese

In a small saucepan, combine the farro and water. Bring to a simmer. Stir once, and then cook for about 15 minutes, until the farro is just cooked through but still has some bite. Drain the farro and transfer it to a medium serving bowl.

Meanwhile, warm the oil in a medium nonstick skillet over medium heat. Add the asparagus and stir-fry for 2 minutes. Add the peas and stir-fry for another 2 minutes, until the vegetables are crisp-tender. Remove the skillet from the heat. Stir in the scallions, parsley, lemon zest, and lemon juice.

Add the asparagus mixture to the farro in the bowl and toss to blend. Season to taste with salt and pepper.

Top each serving with half the ricotta.

NUTRITION INFO: *330 calories, 22 grams protein, 56 grams carbs, 11 grams fiber, 7 grams fat*

STEAK AND RATATOUILLE STIR-FRY

Serves 2

Ratatouille is a Mediterranean dish of eggplant, zucchini, bell peppers, and tomatoes. In late summer, when vegetables are at their freshest, it's particularly delicious. To facilitate cutting the meat into thin slices, put it in the freezer for 10 minutes.

INGREDIENTS

1 teaspoon olive oil

4 ounces top round beef steak, thinly sliced

Salt and black pepper

½ small eggplant, chopped into ¾-inch dice

½ medium zucchini, chopped into ½-inch dice

½ red bell pepper, diced

1 cup diced canned tomatoes with juice

1 clove garlic, minced

1 tablespoon prepared pesto sauce

1 teaspoon red wine vinegar

1 cup cooked brown rice

Warm the oil in a medium cast-iron or heavy skillet over medium heat. Season the beef with salt and pepper, spread it in an even layer in the hot skillet, and cook for 1 minute without stirring. Flip the slices over and cook for 1 minute, until browned, stirring. Using tongs, transfer the steak to a bowl.

Add the eggplant, zucchini, bell pepper, tomatoes, and garlic to the pan. Reduce the heat to medium-low and cook for 10 minutes, stirring often, until the vegetables are softened. Stir in the pesto, vinegar, and cooked beef; cook for 1 minute to warm through.

Meanwhile, warm the rice in the microwave. Divide the rice into two serving bowls and top it with ratatouille.

NUTRITION INFO: *330 calories, 24 grams protein, 36 grams carbs, 9 grams fiber, 12 grams fat*

SNACKS

LITE FRENCH TOAST

Serves 2

You can buy separated egg whites in the dairy department. If you don't have a toaster oven, simply broil the toast in a tray placed on an oven rack on the lowest level. Watch carefully so the toast doesn't burn.

INGREDIENTS

8 egg whites (or 1 cup egg whites)   Cooking spray

1 teaspoon ground cinnamon   3 slices high-fiber bread

Whisk together the egg whites and cinnamon in a bowl.

Coat the tray of the toaster oven with cooking spray.

Place the bread on the toaster tray, cover with the egg white mixture, and toast until the bread is crunchy and the egg whites are set.

NUTRITION INFO: *186 calories, 19 grams protein, 27 grams carbs, 5 grams fiber, 0 grams fat*

BELL PEPPER AND TURKEY ROLL-UPS

Serves 1

You can make these roll-ups ahead of time, wrap them in plastic wrap, and refrigerate.

INGREDIENTS

2 slices deli-style turkey breast

½ cup sliced red bell pepper

1 tablespoon whole-grain mustard

Place the turkey slices on a cutting board and spread mustard on them. Lay the red bell pepper slices on top.

Roll tightly and secure each with a toothpick.

NUTRITION INFO: *134 calories, 26 grams protein, 3 grams carbs, 1 gram fiber, 2 grams fat*

RED LENTIL PUREE

Serves 4

This hearty dip will keep for up to a week refrigerated. Serve warm or at room temperature.

INGREDIENTS

1 cup red lentils, washed and picked over

1 cup reduced-sodium chicken broth

3 tablespoons lemon juice

1 teaspoon chopped fresh thyme or ½ teaspoon dried

Salt and black pepper

Celery stalks, for dipping

In a small saucepan over medium-high heat, combine the lentils and broth, and bring to a boil. Reduce the heat to low, cover, and simmer for 12 minutes, until the lentils have softened. Drain the lentils.

In a food processor, combine the lentils, lemon juice, and thyme. Season with salt and pepper to taste. Process until smooth.

Serve with celery stalks.

NUTRITION INFO: *190 calories, 15 grams protein, 31 grams carbs, 8 grams fiber, 2 grams fat*

PEAR CRUMBLE WITH GREEK YOGURT

Serves 4

Be sure to use plain Greek yogurt, not one with added sugar or pre-serves. Pears and cinnamon give this snack all the sweetness it needs. Substitute apples or berries if you wish, though note that the berries will cook faster.

INGREDIENTS

2 medium pears (any kind), cored and sliced

2 teaspoons ground cinnamon

4 tablespoons Grape-Nuts

2 cups nonfat plain Greek yogurt

Preheat the oven to 375°F.

Fill an 8-inch-square glass baking dish with water to a depth of ¾ inch. Place the sliced pears in the baking dish and sprinkle them with the cinnamon.

Bake for 15 minutes, then reduce the heat to 200°F. Sprinkle with the Grape-Nuts and bake until the pears are the desired softness, an additional 10 to 20 minutes.

To serve, divide the yogurt into four bowls. Place one-quarter of the pear-cereal mix in each bowl, and drizzle with 2 to 3 tablespoons of the warm pan liquid.

NUTRITION INFO: *140 calories, 11 grams protein, 26 grams carbs, 4 grams fiber, 0 grams fat*

SKINNY GUACAMOLE

Serves 4

Substitute cooked, shelled edamame for the peas if you wish. Hass avocados are the dark green or black ones with a bumpy skin, unlike the smooth-skinned bright green type. Seed the chile pepper if you prefer less heat.

INGREDIENTS

1 cup frozen peas, slightly thawed

1 medium Hass avocado, peeled

2 tablespoons lime juice

1 medium tomato

¼ red or sweet onion

1 jalapeño or serrano chile pepper

3 tablespoons fresh cilantro

1 clove garlic

½ teaspoon salt

¼ teaspoon black pepper

8 Finn Crisp crackers

Place the peas, avocado, lime juice, tomato, onion, chile, cilantro, garlic, salt, and pepper in a blender and pulse until smooth.

Serve with the crackers.

NUTRITION INFO: *167 calories, 4 grams protein, 27 grams carbs, 6 grams fiber, 6 grams fat*

CHOCOLATE-AVOCADO MOUSSE WITH RASPBERRIES

Serves 4

This mousse gets its decadent creaminess from a surprising source—avocado—for a perfect spin on a classic dish. Use the best-quality cocoa powder you can find. It will make a difference in the taste. Coconut sugar is available in natural foods stores. If raspberries aren't in season, garnish with mint sprigs if you wish.

INGREDIENTS

2 tablespoons semisweet chocolate chips

1 very ripe Hass avocado, peeled

2 tablespoons unsweetened cocoa powder

2 tablespoons coconut sugar or sweetener of your choice

¾ teaspoon vanilla extract

Dash of salt or sea salt

2½ tablespoons unsweetened plain almond milk or skim milk

Fresh raspberries for garnish

Melt the chocolate chips in a small bowl placed over a saucepan of simmering water. Stir the chocolate until it's melted and smooth, being careful not to scorch it.

Place the melted chocolate, avocado, cocoa powder, coconut sugar, vanilla, salt, and almond milk in a blender or food processor. Blend on the lowest setting until the mixture is smooth and creamy, stopping a few times to scrape the sides of the container.

Spoon the mixture into four small crack-resistant dishes (Pyrex or ice cream glasses) and refrigerate for at least 1½ hours.

Garnish with raspberries just before serving.

NUTRITION INFO: *140 calories, 2 grams protein, 16 grams carbs, 5 grams fiber, 9 grams fat*

BERRY-MUESLI YOGURT PARFAIT

Serves 1

Familia and Alpen, among other brands, offer muesli without added sugar. If you use frozen berries, thaw them for an hour before serving.

INGREDIENTS

½ cup nonfat plain Greek yogurt

¼ cup blueberries, fresh or frozen

¼ cup raspberries, fresh or frozen

2 tablespoons muesli

Mix or layer the yogurt, blueberries, raspberries, and muesli in a bowl or parfait glass and serve.

NUTRITION INFO: *133 calories, 12 grams protein, 22 grams carbs, 4 grams fiber, 1 gram fat*

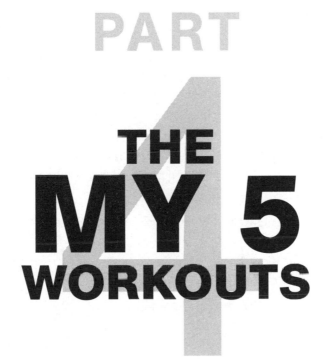

PART 4

THE MY 5
WORKOUTS

GET STARTED

As a reminder, you'll do one exercise each day, for about 5 minutes, following a brief warmup. The program is adaptable to every level of fitness, from Beginner to Advanced, and is designed to allow you make modifications and add variety as you build your strength and endurance in a number of ways. You may want to review Chapter 2 before beginning. Over 7 days, you'll work every major muscle group. On Day 8, repeat this sequence of exercises. Continue to perform one exercise daily for a total of 6 weeks, moving from Beginner (if necessary) to Intermediate and finally Advanced. If you have not yet moved to Advanced after 6 weeks, wait until you do so before moving to the next group of seven daily exercises starting on page 224.

	WHICH EXERCISES	HOW LONG	COMMENTS
Get Started	Basic Exercises	6 weeks	On Day 8, repeat series of 7 exercises for the next week, and so forth.
Add Variety	Alternate Exercises	6 weeks	In the first week, perform the 7 alternate exercises, one per day. In Week 2, revert to the 7 basic exercises. Repeat this sequence for at least 6 weeks and have reached the Advanced level.
Take It Up a Notch	Paired Exercises	Indefinitely	Perform 2 exercises each day, moving from Intermediate to Advanced as your muscles strengthen.

DAY 1 REVERSE LUNGE

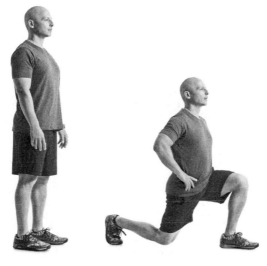

MUSCLE GROUPS WORKED: Quads, hamstrings, and butt (glutes)

FYI: There are many variations of lunges. I like a reverse lunge as an introductory lunge because it's simple and reduces strain on the knees.

HOW TO DO IT:

Start by standing upright, feet shoulder-width apart, and take a large controlled step backward with your right leg. Lower your hips so that your front thigh is parallel to the floor and your left knee is directly over your ankle. Keep your right knee bent at a 90-degree angle and pointing toward the floor. Keep your back straight and look straight ahead.

When your right knee is almost (but not actually) touching the floor, contract your left thigh to return your right leg back to starting position. Repeat with left leg. That's one rep.

BEGINNER: Complete 10 reps. Rest 1 minute. Then repeat 2 more sets of 10 reps with another 1-minute rest between sets.

INTERMEDIATE: Complete 20 reps. Rest 1 minute. Then repeat 2 more sets of 20 reps with another 1-minute rest between sets.

ADVANCED: Complete 30 reps. Rest 1 minute. Then repeat 2 more sets of 30 reps with another 1-minute rest between sets.

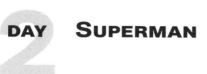

DAY 2 SUPERMAN

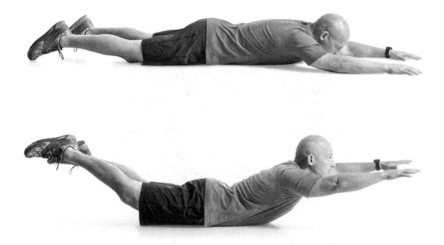

MUSCLE GROUPS WORKED: Lower back (spinal erectors) and butt (glutes) and some hamstring

FYI: Superman helps create a long, flat midsection by strengthening the lower back.

HOW TO DO IT:

Lie with your face down on the floor and your arms and legs fully extended so that your body looks like the letter X from above.

From this position, lift your arms/chest and thighs toward the ceiling as though you were flying, and then lower them down to the beginning position. Do not hold the pose; just keep going up and down without resting on the floor.

BEGINNER: Complete 10 reps. Rest 1 minute. Then repeat 2 more sets of 10 reps with another 1-minute rest between sets.

INTERMEDIATE: Complete 20 reps. Rest 1 minute. Then repeat 2 more sets of 20 reps with another 1-minute rest between sets.

ADVANCED: Complete 30 reps. Rest 1 minute. Then repeat 2 more sets of 30 reps with another 1-minute rest between sets.

DAY 3 LYING DUMBBELL TRICEPS EXTENSION

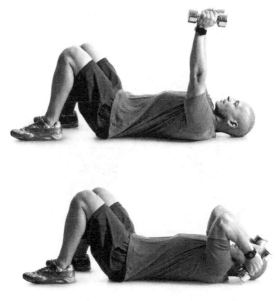

MUSCLE GROUPS WORKED: Triceps

FYI: Your triceps are the muscles that run along the back of your upper arm. Most people overexercise their biceps and underexercise their triceps.

HOW TO DO IT:

Lying on your back, hold a dumbbell in each hand with your arms fully extended toward the ceiling, your palms facing each other. Hinging at your elbows, lower the dumbbells until they are next to your ears. (Don't let them touch the floor.)

Then extend toward the ceiling, returning to starting position.

BEGINNER: Complete 10 reps. Rest 1 minute. Then repeat 2 more sets of 10 reps with another 1-minute rest between sets.

INTERMEDIATE: Complete 20 reps. Rest 1 minute. Then repeat 2 more sets of 20 reps with another 1-minute rest between sets.

ADVANCED: Complete 30 reps. Rest 1 minute. Then repeat 2 more sets of 30 reps with another 1-minute rest between sets.

DAY STIFF-LEG DUMBBELL DEADLIFT

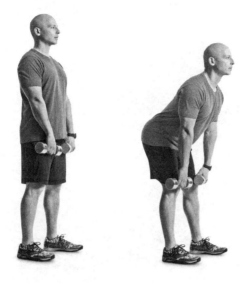

MUSCLE GROUPS WORKED: Hamstrings, glutes

FYI: This is a great exercise for working your hamstrings and butt.

HOW TO DO IT:

Stand with your feet about shoulder-width apart, with a dumbbell in each hand in front of you, palms facing in toward the front of your thighs.

Inhale and, while hinging at the hips but keeping your back arched, push your butt backward and slide the dumbbells down the front of your thighs. Push your hips back as far as you can, feeling a stretch in your hamstrings.

When you can no longer push your hips any farther back, inhale while sliding your hips forward, back to standing. Repeat.

BEGINNER: Complete 10 reps. Rest 1 minute. Then repeat 2 more sets of 10 reps with another 1-minute rest between sets.

INTERMEDIATE: Complete 20 reps. Rest 1 minute. Then repeat 2 more sets of 20 reps with another 1-minute rest between sets.

ADVANCED: Complete 30 reps. Rest 1 minute. Then repeat 2 more sets of 30 reps with another 1-minute rest between sets.

DAY STANDING DUMBBELL CURL PRESS

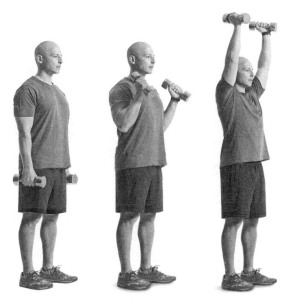

MUSCLE GROUPS WORKED: Biceps and shoulders

FYI: This is a compound movement and combines a biceps curl with a shoulder press, efficiently targeting two areas at once.

HOW TO DO IT:

Hold a dumbbell in each hand with your palms facing toward your body.

Slowly curl the dumbbells up toward your shoulders, and then continue to press them up toward the ceiling.

Do the same in reverse as you lower the dumbbells down to starting position.

BEGINNER: Complete 10 reps. Rest 1 minute. Then repeat 2 more sets of 10 reps with another 1-minute rest between sets.

INTERMEDIATE: Complete 20 reps. Rest 1 minute. Then repeat 2 more sets of 20 reps with another 1-minute rest between sets.

ADVANCED: Complete 30 reps. Rest 1 minute. Then repeat 2 more sets of 30 reps with another 1-minute rest between sets.

DAY SINGLE-ARM DUMBBELL ROW

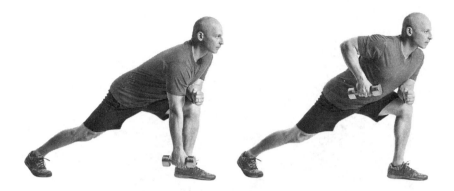

MUSCLE GROUPS WORKED: Upper back (rhomboid and lower trapezius), rear shoulders, and biceps

FYI: This exercise is great for your upper-body posture. Imagine that you're starting a lawn mower as you pull back. Use only one dumbbell at a time.

HOW TO DO IT:

Start in a lunge position with your left knee forward and your right leg extended all the way back. Hold the dumbbell in your right hand with your arm extended down. Place your left forearm across your left thigh for support, and pull the dumbbell back with your right arm in a slow, controlled movement. Make sure to "drag" your elbow along your ribs and across your body on the way up.

Return to starting position.

Repeat with right knee forward and the left leg extended all the way back, holding the dumbbell in your left hand.

BEGINNER: Complete 10 reps on each side. Rest 1 minute. Then repeat 2 more sets of 10 reps per side with another 1-minute rest between sets.

INTERMEDIATE: Complete 20 reps on each side. Rest 1 minute. Then repeat 2 more sets of 20 reps on each side with another 1-minute rest between sets.

ADVANCED: Complete 30 reps on each side. Rest 1 minute. Then repeat 2 more sets of 30 reps on each side with another 1-minute rest between sets.

DAY 7

STANDING DUMBBELL SIDE BEND

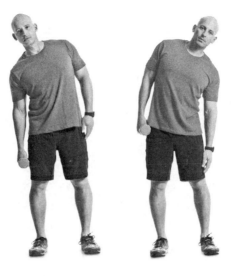

MUSCLE GROUPS WORKED: External and internal obliques (a.k.a. "love handles")

FYI: These movements will not only tone your sides but also help carve the inguinal (the sexy lines that go from your hip to your groin).

HOW TO DO IT:

Stand straight with your feet shoulder-width apart, holding a dumbbell in your left hand. Gently tilt your upper body to the right as you stretch your left "love handles." Return to starting position, and repeat.

Then reverse direction as you slide the dumbbell down your left thigh and stretch out your right side.

BEGINNER: Complete 10 reps on either side. Rest 1 minute. Then repeat 2 more sets of 10 reps on either side with another 1-minute rest between sets.

INTERMEDIATE: Complete 20 reps on either side. Rest 1 minute. Then repeat 2 more sets of 20 reps on either side with another 1-minute rest between sets.

ADVANCED: Complete 30 reps on either side. Rest 1 minute. Then repeat 2 more sets of 30 reps on either side with another 1-minute rest between sets.

ADD VARIETY

After 2 weeks of doing the basic exercises, you can begin to alternate the seven moves on the following pages with the ones you've been doing. Do these new moves one week and the following week go back to the original moves, and so forth, for a minimum of 6 weeks . What's the reasoning behind this change? As I've explained earlier, boredom can interfere with your commitment to your resistance exercise program. Plus once an exercise is too easy, its benefit decreases. The following seven exercises work the same muscles, but in slightly different ways, adding to both the challenge and enhancing the benefit. After 6 weeks, if you have moved up to the Advanced level, it's time to move to the paired exercises starting on page 232.

DAY SINGLE-LEG TAP SQUAT

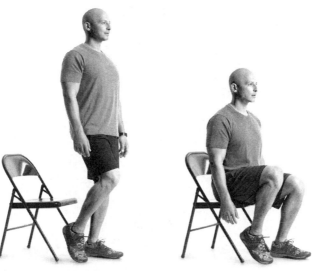

INSTEAD OF: Reverse Lunge

MUSCLE GROUPS WORKED: Front of the thighs (quads) and glutes

FYI: The move helps develop your balance as well as your strength. Rather than just sitting straight down, be sure to move your hips backward and down.

HOW TO DO IT:

Stand in front of a bench or chair. Shift your weight to your left leg, lift your right leg off the ground, and lower your body until your butt just taps the top front of the bench or chair.

Immediately come back up to starting position and repeat.

Repeat, supporting yourself on your right leg and lifting your left leg off the ground.

BEGINNER: Complete 10 reps on each leg. Rest 1 minute. Then repeat 2 more sets of 10 reps per leg with another 1-minute rest between sets.

INTERMEDIATE: Complete 20 reps on each leg. Rest 1 minute. Then repeat 2 more sets of 20 reps on each leg with another 1-minute rest between sets.

ADVANCED: Complete 30 reps on each leg. Rest 1 minute. Then repeat 2 more sets of 30 reps on each leg with another 1-minute rest between sets.

DAY 2 HIP THRUST

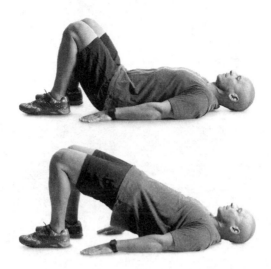

INSTEAD OF: Superman

MUSCLE GROUPS WORKED: Spinal erectors (lower back) and glutes

FYI: This exercise helps lengthen your midsection by strengthening your lower back and glutes. To add intensity, hold the lifted position longer or add some weight to the top of your pelvis.

HOW TO DO IT:

Lie on the floor or an exercise mat with your head, neck, and back flat so your spine is in one straight line. Bend your knees so that your feet are also flat on the ground, shoulder-width apart and parallel. Exhale and, using your lower back and glutes, drive your butt off the floor until your head, hips, and knees are in line.

Slowly lower your hips and buttocks back down to starting position, and repeat.

BEGINNER: Complete 10 reps. Rest 1 minute. Then repeat 2 more sets of 10 reps with another 1-minute rest between sets.

INTERMEDIATE: Complete 20 reps. Rest 1 minute. Then repeat 2 more sets of 20 reps with another 1-minute rest between sets.

ADVANCED: Complete 30 reps. Rest 1 minute. Then repeat 2 more sets of 30 reps with another 1-minute rest between sets.

DAY **DUMBBELL SINGLE-ARM TRICEPS KICKBACK**

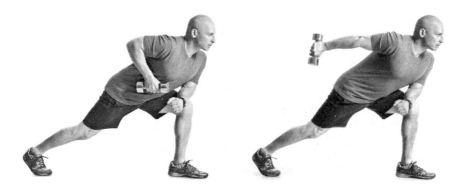

INSTEAD OF: Lying Dumbbell Triceps Extension

MUSCLE GROUPS WORKED: Triceps

FYI: The back of the arm is often a trouble spot for women, but it's also the key to having great upper arms.

HOW TO DO IT:

Using a staggered stance with your left leg forward, place your left hand on your left thigh for support. With a dumbbell in hand, hinge from your elbow and extend your right forearm back until it's parallel with the floor.

Return to starting position, keeping the elbow hinged, and repeat.

Repeat with your right leg forward, extending your left arm.

BEGINNER: Complete 10 reps on each arm. Rest 1 minute. Then repeat 2 more sets of 10 reps per arm with another 1-minute rest between sets.

INTERMEDIATE: Complete 20 reps on each arm. Rest 1 minute. Then repeat 2 more sets of 20 reps on per arm with another 1-minute rest between sets.

ADVANCED: Complete 30 reps on each arm. Rest 1 minute. Then repeat 2 more sets of 30 reps on per arm with another 1-minute rest between sets.

DAY 4 — BALL HAMSTRING CURL

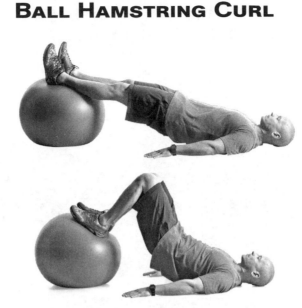

INSTEAD OF: Stiff-Leg Dumbbell Deadlift

MUSCLE GROUPS WORKED: Hamstrings

FYI: You'll need a stability ball to do this exercise. Make sure it is the proper size—they range from 55 to 65 inches in circumference—for your height.

HOW TO DO IT:

Lie on your back with your arms flat on the floor at your sides, palms down, and rest your heels on top of an exercise ball. Press your heels down onto the ball.

Slowly raise your hips up and bend your knees, rolling the ball slightly toward your butt as far as you can. Pause and roll the ball back by straightening your legs. Make sure you keep your hips as high as you can off the floor throughout the set. Repeat.

BEGINNER: Complete 10 reps. Rest 1 minute. Then repeat 2 more sets of 10 reps with another 1-minute rest between sets.

INTERMEDIATE: Complete 20 reps. Rest 1 minute. Then repeat 2 more sets of 20 reps with another 1-minute rest between sets.

ADVANCED: Complete 30 reps. Rest 1 minute. Then repeat 2 more sets of 30 reps with another 1-minute rest between sets.

DUMBBELL LATERAL RAISE

DAY 5

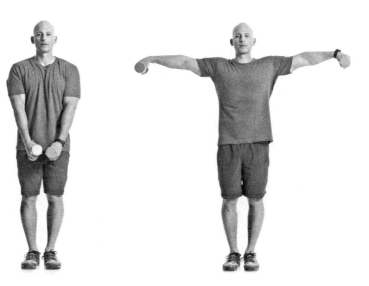

INSTEAD OF: Standing Dumbbell Curl Press

MUSCLE GROUPS WORKED: Shoulders

FYI: As you do this exercise, imagine you're a puppet with strings attached to your wrists that someone is pulling up.

HOW TO DO IT:

Stand up straight with your feet hip-width apart and with a dumbbell in each hand. Your arms should be hanging in front of your thighs with slight bend in the elbow and palms facing each other. Engage your shoulders by raising your arms to shoulder height to either side until they're parallel to the ground. Make sure you keep your wrists limp throughout the set.

Slowly return your arms to your sides, and repeat.

BEGINNER: Complete 10 reps. Rest 1 minute. Then repeat 2 more sets of 10 reps with another 1-minute rest between sets.

INTERMEDIATE: Complete 20 reps. Rest 1 minute. Then repeat 2 more sets of 20 reps with another 1-minute rest between sets.

ADVANCED: Complete 30 reps. Rest 1 minute. Then repeat 2 more sets of 30 reps with another 1-minute rest between sets.

DAY 6 REVERSE FLY

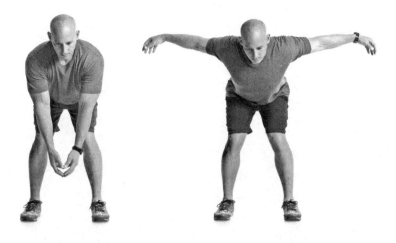

INSTEAD OF: Single-Arm Dumbbell Row

MUSCLE GROUPS WORKED: Upper back and shoulders

FYI: This exercise sculpts a strong, sexy back. As you do it, imagine that you are flying away—think of your arms as long wings. Keep a slight bend in your elbows throughout the exercise. Feel free to add dumbbells as you advance.

HOW TO DO IT:

Stand with your feet shoulder-width apart. Stick your butt out and lean forward until your upper torso is parallel to the floor. Raise your hands out at your sides. Stop when your arms are parallel to the floor and squeeze your shoulder blades together at the top of the movement. Keep your wrists limp throughout the set.

Slowly lower your arms back down toward your sides, and repeat.

BEGINNER: Complete 10 reps. Rest 1 minute. Then repeat 2 more sets of 10 reps with another 1-minute rest between sets.

INTERMEDIATE: Complete 20 reps. Rest 1 minute. Then repeat 2 more sets of 20 reps with another 1-minute rest between sets.

ADVANCED: Complete 30 reps. Rest 1 minute. Then repeat 2 more sets of 30 reps with another 1-minute rest between sets.

DAY 7   SIDE PLANK

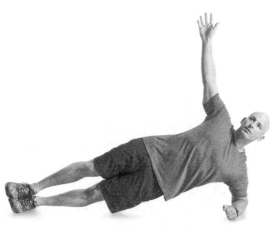

INSTEAD OF: Standing Dumbbell Side Bend

MUSCLE GROUPS WORKED: Obliques; also chest, back, and core abdominal muscles

FYI: This move helps whittle your waist and banish your "love handles."

HOW TO DO IT:

Lie on your right side on the floor or a mat, placing your forearm in front of yourself and stacking your feet one upon the other. Exhale and raise your body, supporting it on your forearm and feet. Inhale, and contract your abdominal muscles. Hold for 30/45/60 seconds, depending upon your skill level.

Return to starting position, and repeat.

Repeat, lying on your left side.

BEGINNER: Hold 30 seconds on each side. Rest 1 minute. Then repeat 2 more holds of 30 seconds per side with another 1-minute rest between holds.

INTERMEDIATE: Hold 45 seconds on each side. Rest 1 minute. Then repeat 2 more holds of 45 seconds on each side with another 1-minute rest between holds.

ADVANCED: Hold 60 seconds on each side. Rest 1 minute. Then repeat 2 more holds of 60 seconds on each side with another 1-minute rest between holds.

TAKE IT UP A NOTCH

Once you've reached the Advanced level of Add Variety and have spent a minimum of 6 weeks alternating the new exercises with the basic ones, you're ready to take your fitness program to the next level, combining two exercises each day. Your new moves appear on the following pages. Some pairs include two exercises you've already mastered, others pair a new move with an old one, and two pair a couple new exercises. You'll now be spending about 10 minutes a day on your workout. Starting with one exercise, complete 1 set, whether that includes 10, 20, or 30 reps. Rest for 1 minute, and then complete 1 set of the second exercise. Rest for 1 minute and repeat the first exercise and so forth. Your objective is to complete 3 sets of both exercises with 1-minute rests between the second and third sets of each move. You may find initially that you can complete fewer reps for one or both exercises than you had been doing earlier. Perhaps you'll need to drop back to the Intermediate level. Or you may want to drop back to Beginner for a week to familiarize yourself with the new set of seven daily exercises before moving to Intermediate and finally Advanced.

DAY 1 PIKE PLANK

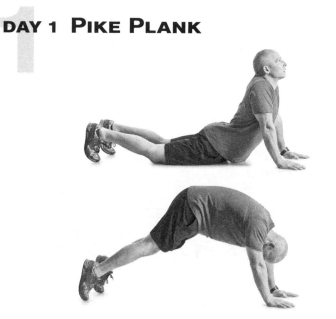

PAIR WITH: Reverse Lunge (page 217)

MUSCLE GROUPS WORKED: Rectus abdominals (the front of the midsection), quads, and glutes

FYI: I love this exercise because it stretches the abs and lower back between every repetition.

HOW TO DO IT:

Lie on the floor or a mat with your palms flat on the floor directly beneath your shoulders and your lower legs resting on the floor with your toes tucked in toward your body, and look up. Pulling your abs in, raise your pelvis straight up, supported by your hands, and look at the laces on your shoes.

Raise the rest of your body, looking down; then return to starting position, and repeat.

BEGINNER: Complete 10 reps. Rest 1 minute. Then repeat 2 more sets of 10 reps with another 1-minute rest between sets.

INTERMEDIATE: Complete 20 reps. Rest 1 minute. Then repeat 2 more sets of 20 reps with another 1-minute rest between sets.

ADVANCED: Complete 30 reps. Rest 1 minute. Then repeat 2 more sets of 30 reps with another 1-minute rest between sets.

DAY 2   ## LYING DUMBBELL TRICEPS EXTENSION (PAGE 219)

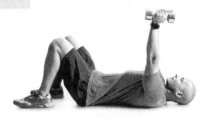

PAIR WITH: Hip Thrust (page 226)

MUSCLE GROUPS WORKED: Triceps, lower back, and glutes

DAY 3   ## STANDING DUMBBELL SIDE BEND (PAGE 223)

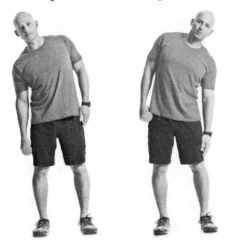

PAIR WITH: Stiff-Leg Dumbbell Deadlift (page 220)

MUSCLE GROUPS WORKED: Hamstrings and obliques

DAY 4 SEATED TRUNK TWIST

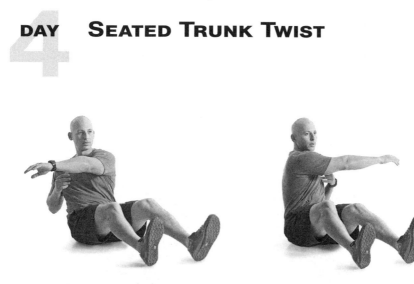

PAIR WITH: Standing Dumbbell Shoulder Press (page 236)

MUSCLE GROUPS WORKED: Transverse abs (corset muscles) and obliques

FYI: The corset muscle wraps all the way around your midsection. If strengthened properly, these muscles can help "pull" your tummy in. The movement is relatively slight. Be sure to move only your upper body, not your hips.

HOW TO DO IT:

Sit on the floor or on an exercise mat with your legs extended and slightly bent and only your heels touching the floor. Lean slightly back. Extend your left arm at shoulder height and slowly rotate your arm and rib cage to the right, as though reaching for the right wall while contracting your tummy. Then repeat with your right arm extended and slowly rotating your arm and rib cage to the left, again contracting your tummy.

Repeat, alternating from a left twist to a right twist.

BEGINNER: Complete 20 reps on each side. Rest 1 minute. Then repeat 2 more sets of 20 reps per side with another 1-minute rest between sets.

INTERMEDIATE: Complete 30 reps on each side. Rest 1 minute. Then repeat 2 more sets of 30 reps on each side with another 1-minute rest between sets.

ADVANCED: Complete 40 reps on each side. Rest 1 minute. Then repeat 2 more sets of 40 reps on each side with another 1-minute rest between sets.

DAY 4   PAIR WITH: STANDING DUMBBELL SHOULDER PRESS

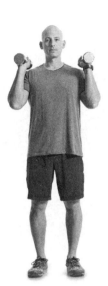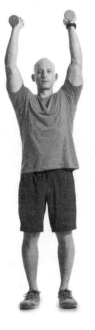

MUSCLE GROUPS WORKED: Shoulders and triceps

FYI: Be sure to keep your knees slightly bent to protect your lower back.

HOW TO DO IT:

Hold the dumbbells at shoulder level with palms facing in and elbows bent. Keeping your back straight, slowly raise the dumbbells overhead until your arms are fully extended.

Slowly return to starting position. Repeat.

BEGINNER: Complete 10 reps. Rest 1 minute. Then repeat 2 more sets of 10 reps with another 1-minute rest between sets.

INTERMEDIATE: Complete 20 reps. Rest 1 minute. Then repeat 2 more sets of 20 reps with another 1-minute rest between sets.

ADVANCED: Complete 30 reps. Rest 1 minute. Then repeat 2 more sets of 30 reps with another 1-minute rest between sets.

DAY 5 | SINGLE-ARM DUMBBELL ROW (PAGE 222)

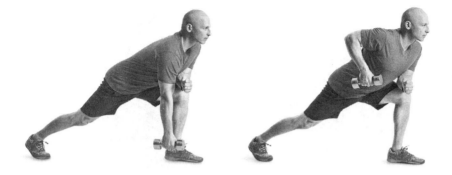

PAIR WITH: Superman (page 218)

MUSCLE GROUPS WORKED: Rhomboids (upper back) and lower back

DAY DUMBBELL HAMMER BICEPS CURL

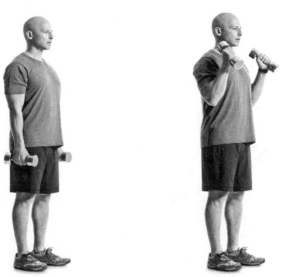

PAIR WITH: Plank (opposite)

MUSCLE GROUPS WORKED: Biceps and rectus abs

FYI: Hinge from your elbows and keep your arms pinned to your sides. Nothing should move from your shoulders to your elbows.

HOW TO DO IT:

Standing with your feet hip-width apart, grasp a dumbbell in each hand with your arms extended downward and your palms facing inward. Keeping your upper arms pressed against your rib cage, exhale as you hinge at the elbows and bring each head of the dumbbell up toward your shoulders.

Inhale as you return to starting position, and repeat.

BEGINNER: Complete 10 reps. Rest 1 minute. Then repeat 2 more sets of 10 reps with another 1-minute rest between sets.

INTERMEDIATE: Complete 20 reps. Rest 1 minute. Then repeat 2 more sets of 20 reps with another 1-minute rest between sets.

ADVANCED: Complete 30 reps. Rest 1 minute. Then repeat 2 more sets of 30 reps with another 1-minute rest between sets.

DAY 6 PLANK

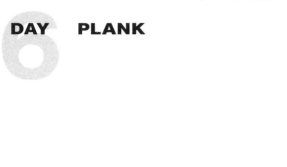

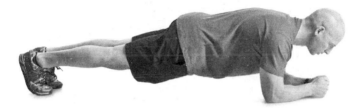

MUSCLE GROUPS WORKED: Rectus abdominals (front of your core)

FYI: A more advanced plank involves raising one leg, which creates instability, making your abs work harder.

HOW TO DO IT:

Rest your forearms on the floor and extend your legs back so your toes are on the ground and there's a straight line from your heels to your shoulders. Contract your midsection, forming a rigid plank with your body, and hold as long as you can. Make sure you breathe!

BEGINNER: Hold for 30 seconds. Rest 1 minute. Then repeat twice with another 1-minute rest between the two.

INTERMEDIATE: Hold for 45 seconds. Rest 1 minute. Then repeat twice with another 1-minute rest between the two.

ADVANCED: Hold for 60 seconds. Rest 1 minute. Then repeat twice with another 1-minute rest between the two.

DAY 7   LYING TRUNK TWIST

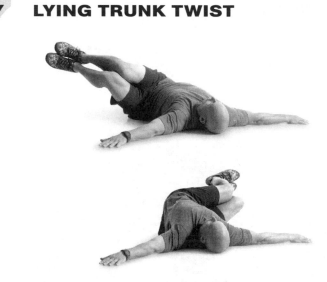

PAIR WITH: Sumo Squat or Pushup (men only)

MUSCLE GROUPS WORKED: Transverse abs (corset muscle) and obliques

FYI: Unlike the Seated Trunk Twist, in which you move your upper body, this exercise moves your lower body, which is why it's also known as a lower body trunk twist. It strengthens the corset and actually "pulls in" your midsection.

HOW TO DO IT:

Lie on your back on the floor or an exercise mat with your legs in the air and knees bent at a 90-degree angle directly over your hips. Keeping your shoulders flat on the floor and arms straight out to the sides, with your palms facing up, and holding your legs together, rotate your lower body to the left side until your left leg touches (or comes close to) the floor.

Then rotate your lower body to the opposite side, until your right legs touches the floor. That's one rep.

BEGINNER: Complete 15 reps. Rest 1 minute. Then repeat 2 more sets of 15 reps with another 1-minute rest between sets.

INTERMEDIATE: Complete 20 reps. Rest 1 minute. Then repeat 2 more sets of 20 reps with another 1-minute rest between sets.

ADVANCED: Complete 25 reps on each side. Rest 1 minute. Then repeat 2 more sets of 25 reps with another 1-minute rest between sets.

DAY 7 SUMO SQUAT

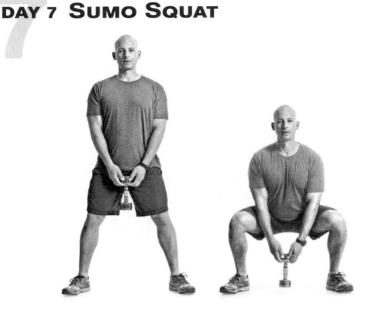

MUSCLE GROUPS WORKED: Inner thigh, glutes, and quads

FYI: These squats are so named because they mimic the position used by sumo wrestlers.

HOW TO DO IT:

Stand holding the end of one dumbbell with both hands, arms in front of your belly and extended toward the floor; place your feet more than hip-width apart, with your toes turned out slightly and your knees soft.

Slowly bend your knees, lowering your butt until your knees are at about a 90-degree angle, keeping your chest up to reduce back strain. Pause, press through your heels, and return to starting position; repeat.

BEGINNER: Complete 10 reps. Rest 1 minute. Then repeat 2 more sets of 10 reps with another 1-minute rest between sets.

INTERMEDIATE: Complete 20 reps. Rest 1 minute. Then repeat 2 more sets of 20 reps with another 1-minute rest between sets.

ADVANCED: Complete 30 reps. Rest 1 minute. Then repeat 2 more sets of 30 reps with another 1-minute rest between sets.

DAY PUSHUP (MEN ONLY)

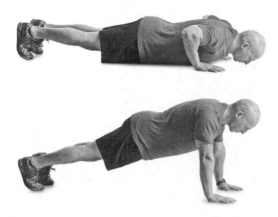

MUSCLE GROUPS WORKED: Chest, shoulders, and triceps

FYI: This is not an exercise for beginners and can interfere with good posture by over-strengthening the front of the body. Gals, instead, do the Sumo Squat on page 241.

HOW TO DO IT:

Lie on your stomach on the floor or a mat with your legs stretched out behind you, feet flexed, and toes pointed toward the ground. Place your palms down, slightly more than shoulder-width apart. Looking at the floor, straighten your arms and push your entire body up so that only your hands and toes are touching the floor. Keep your palms fixed in the same position and keep your body straight and stiff. Don't arch your back or let your stomach sag toward the floor. Exhale as your arms straighten, and pause at the top, when your arms are nearly straight.

Inhale as you bend your arms to lower your body until your chest touches the floor, keeping your knees off the floor, and repeat.

INTERMEDIATE: Complete 20 reps, holding each for a count of 45. Rest 1 minute. Then repeat 2 more sets of 20 reps with another 1-minute rest between sets.

ADVANCED: Complete 30 reps, holding each for a count of 60. Rest 1 minute. Then repeat 2 more sets of 30 reps with another 1-minute rest between sets.

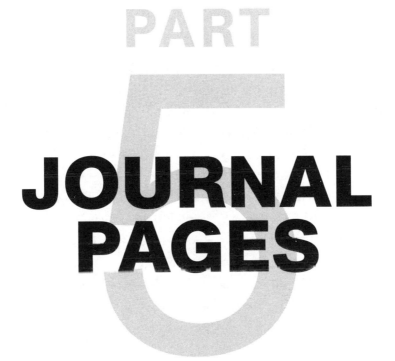

PART 5

JOURNAL PAGES

WRITE IT DOWN!

Answer each question with a yes or no. When you're just starting out, it will be helpful to add some commentary, particularly if you answer no to a question. Be straightforward (only you will see this), explaining what stood between you and a yes answer. Also record your feelings, any challenges you faced, your sense of accomplishment, and the like. It's helpful to add details, such as which foods you ate or how many sets and reps you did of the resistance exercises. After the initial 5 days, as My 5 becomes second nature, you may not need to supply as much detail. My philosophy is that simpler is always better, particularly once you're in the groove. For that reason, the sample journal page that you can photocopy for Day 6 and beyond is less detailed. Bottom line: Follow whatever approach works best for you, whether that's including details or just answering a quick yes or no to the five questions.

You'll notice that I don't ask you to enter either your starting weight or your weight from day to day. That's because, as I explained on page 145, the scale is an unreliable tool since your weight naturally fluctuates from day to day, depending on your body's natural processes—and, if you're a premenopausal woman, upon where you are in your monthly cycle. Either of these factors could create a 4-pound or greater seesaw in weight. A more reliable measure is how a pair of tight jeans fits from day to day. Of course, you're free to enter your weight in this journal if you must, but just don't let it discourage you if your results aren't immediately reflected on the scale.

I've filled in the following sample journal page as an example of the kinds of entries you might make in the first 5 days. Continue to use the journal pages to stay motivated until you achieve your goal and then to maintain your new weight.

DAY 1: ___*3/4/15*___ (date)

Did you eat three meals (protein, fibrous carbs, and healthy fats) and two snacks (protein and fiber) today? Yes _____ No __*X*__

Breakfast: *Egg white scramble, avocado, high-fiber English muffin*

Snack: _____

Lunch: *Cobb salad*

Snack: *High-protein, high-fiber snack bar*

_____

Dinner: *Salmon fillet, green beans, brown rice*

Comments: *Missed my morning snack because I got caught in a meeting that ran to lunchtime. Tomorrow I'll be sure to have a high-protein snack bar on me or in my desk so this doesn't happen again.*

Did you do 5 minutes of resistance exercise today? Yes __*X*__
No _____

Exercise performed: *Reverse lunge*

Comments: *Did 3 sets of 10 reps on each side for a total of 30. Phew! But it really did only take about 5 minutes.*

Did you take at least 10,000 steps today? Yes __*X*__ No _____

Comments: *My fitbit recorded 9,708 steps but I forgot to put it on until after I got up and got the kids fed and dressed, so I'm sure I was well over 10,000. Will put it on first thing tomorrow!*

Did you sleep at least 7 continuous hours last night excluding a brief bathroom break? Yes __X__ No _____

Comments: *I made a real point of getting into bed by 11 last night and slept right through to 6 am, when the baby woke up. felt rested for the first time in months! I'm going to aim for another half hour in the sack tonight. folding laundry can wait until tomorrow!*

Did you unplug (no phone, TV, or computer) for at least 1 hour today?

Yes __X__ No _____

Comments: *This was the hardest thing for me to do. Whenever I'm out of the house, I need to have my phone on so I can always be reached if there's a problem with one of the kids. And Joe and I do like to relax in front of TV for an hour or so after they're in bed. Instead, we sat in front of the fire for an hour before bedtime and talked and read. It was lovely!*

Following are journal pages for each of the first 5 days of My 5 Plan, as well as a page you can photocopy if you decide to continue to keep a journal going forward, as I recommend.

DAY 1: _____ (date)

Did you eat three meals (protein, fibrous carbs, and healthy fats) and two snacks (protein and fiber) today? Yes _____ No _____

Breakfast: _____

Snack: _____

Lunch: _____

_____

Snack: _____

Dinner: _____

Comments: _____

_____

_____

_____

Did you do 5 minutes of resistance exercise today? Yes _____
No _____

Exercise performed: _____

Comments: _____

_____

_____

Did you take at least 10,000 steps today? Yes _____ No _____

Comments:_____

_____

_____

_____

Did you sleep at least 7 continuous hours last night excluding a brief bathroom break? Yes _____ No _____

Comments: _____

_____

_____

_____

_____

Did you unplug (no phone, TV, or computer) for at least 1 hour today?

Yes _____ No _____

Comments: _____

_____

_____

_____

_____

DAY 2: _____ (date)

Did you eat three meals (protein, fibrous carbs, and healthy fats) and two snacks (protein and fiber) today? Yes _____ No _____

Breakfast: _____

Snack: _____

Lunch: _____

_____

Snack: _____

Dinner: _____

Comments: _____

_____

_____

_____

Did you do 5 minutes of resistance exercise today? Yes _____
No _____

Exercise performed: _____

Comments: _____

_____

_____

Did you take at least 10,000 steps today? Yes _____ No _____

Comments: _____

_____

_____

_____

Did you sleep at least 7 continuous hours last night excluding a brief bathroom break? Yes _____ No _____

Comments: _____

_____

_____

_____

_____

Did you unplug (no phone, TV, or computer) for at least 1 hour today?

Yes _____ No _____

Comments: _____

_____

_____

_____

_____

DAY 3: _____ (date)

Did you eat three meals (protein, fibrous carbs, and healthy fats) and two snacks (protein and fiber) today? Yes _____ No _____

Breakfast: _____

Snack: _____

Lunch: _____

_____

Snack: _____

Dinner: _____

Comments: _____

_____

_____

_____

Did you do 5 minutes of resistance exercise today? Yes _____
No _____

Exercise performed: _____

Comments: _____

_____

_____

Did you take at least 10,000 steps today? Yes _____ No _____

Comments:_____

_____

_____

_____

Did you sleep at least 7 continuous hours last night excluding a brief bathroom break? Yes _____ No _____

Comments: _____

_____

_____

_____

_____

Did you unplug (no phone, TV, or computer) for at least 1 hour today?

Yes _____ No _____

Comments: _____

_____

_____

_____

_____

DAY 4: _____ (date)

Did you eat three meals (protein, fibrous carbs, and healthy fats) and two snacks (protein and fiber) today? Yes _____ No _____

Breakfast: _____

Snack: _____

Lunch: _____

_____

Snack: _____

Dinner: _____

Comments: _____

_____

_____

_____

Did you do 5 minutes of resistance exercise today? Yes _____
No _____

Exercise performed: _____

Comments: _____

_____

_____

Did you take at least 10,000 steps today? Yes _____ No _____

Comments:_____

_____

_____

_____

Did you sleep at least 7 continuous hours last night excluding a brief bathroom break? Yes _____ No _____

Comments: _____

_____

_____

_____

_____

Did you unplug (no phone, TV, or computer) for at least 1 hour today?

Yes _____ No _____

Comments: _____

_____

_____

_____

_____

DAY 5: _____ (date)

Did you eat three meals (protein, fibrous carbs, and healthy fats) and two snacks (protein and fiber) today? Yes _____ No _____

Breakfast: _____

Snack: _____

Lunch: _____

_____

Snack: _____

Dinner: _____

Comments: _____

_____

_____

_____

Did you do 5 minutes of resistance exercise today? Yes _____
No _____

Exercise performed: _____

Comments: _____

_____

_____

Did you take at least 10,000 steps today? Yes _____ No _____

Comments:_____

_____

_____

_____

Did you sleep at least 7 continuous hours last night excluding a brief bathroom break? Yes _____ No _____

Comments: _____
_____
_____
_____
_____

Did you unplug (no phone, TV, or computer) for at least 1 hour today?

Yes _____ No _____

Comments: _____
_____
_____
_____
_____

YOU CAN PHOTOCOPY THE FOLLOWING PAGE
TO USE GOING FORWARD.

DATE: _____

Did you eat three meals (protein, fibrous carbs, and healthy fats) and two snacks (protein and fiber) today? Yes _____ No _____

Breakfast: _____

_____

Snack: _____

_____

Lunch: _____

_____

Snack: _____

_____

Dinner: _____

_____

Did you do at least 5 minutes of resistance exercise today?
Yes _____ No _____

Exercise(s) performed: _____

_____

Did you take at least 10,000 steps today? Yes _____ No _____
How many?_____

Did you sleep at least 7 continuous hours last night excluding a brief bathroom break? Yes _____ No _____ How many? _____

Did you unplug (no phone, or TV, computer) for at least 1 hour today? Yes _____ No _____

NOTES

CHAPTER 1: (PROTEIN + FIBER) X 5

1. Jenkins et al. 1995. Effect of nibbling versus gorging on cardiovascular risk factors: Serum uric acid and blood lipids. *Metabolism* 44(4): 549–55.

2. Smith et al. 2012. Daily eating frequency and cardiometabolic risk factors in young Australian adults: Cross-sectional analyses. *British Journal of Nutrition* 108(6): 1086–94.

3. Jenkins et al. 1989. Nibbling versus gorging: Metabolic advantages of increased meal frequency. *New England Journal of Medicine* 321(14): 929–34.

4. Speechly, D.P., and Buffenstein, R. 1999. Greater appetite control associated with an increased frequency of eating in lean males. *Appetite* 33(3): 285–97.

5. Blundell et al. 1993. Dietary fat and the control of energy intake: Evaluating the effects of fat on meal size and post-meal satiety. *American Journal of Clinical Nutrition* 57 (5 Suppl): 772S–8S.

6. Smith et al. 2012. Daily eating frequency and cardiometabolic risk factors in young Australian adults: Cross-sectional analyses. *British Journal of Nutrition* 108(6): 1086–94.

7. Westerterp-Plantenga et al. 2002. Habitual meal frequency and energy intake regulation in partially temporally isolated men. *International Journal of Obesity and Related Metabolic Disorders* 26(1): 102–10.

8. Burley et al. 1993. Influence of a high-fibre food (myco-protein) on appetite: Effects on satiation (within meals) and satiety (following meals). *European Journal of Clinical Nutrition* 47(6): 409–18.

9. La Bounty et al. 2011. International Society of Sports Nutrition position stand: Meal frequency. *Journal of the International Society of Sports Nutrition* 8:4.

10. Gómez-Martínez et al. 2012. Eating habits and total and abdominal fat in Spanish adolescents: Influence of physical activity—the AVENA study. *Journal of Adolescent Health* 50(4): 403–9.

11. Kirk, T.R. 2000. Role of dietary carbohydrate and frequent eating in body-weight control. *Proceedings of the Nutrition Society* 59(3): 349–58.

12. Westerterp-Plantenga et al. 2002. Habitual meal frequency and energy intake regulation in partially temporally isolated men. *International Journal of Obesity and Related Metabolic Disorders* 26(1): 102–110.

13. Gómez-Martínez et al. 2012. Eating habits and total and abdominal fat in Spanish adolescents: influence of physical activity—the AVENA study. *Journal of Adolescent Health* 50(4): 403–9.

14. Metzner et al. 1977. The relationship between frequency of eating and adiposity in adult men and women in the Tecumseh Community Health Study. *American Journal of Clinical Nutrition* 30(5): 712–15.

15. Bachman et al. 2011. Eating frequency is higher in weight-loss maintainers and normal-weight individuals than in overweight individuals. *Journal of the American Dietetic Association* 111(11): 1730–34.

16. La Bounty et al. 2011. International Society of Sports Nutrition position stand: Meal frequency. *Journal of the International Society of Sports Nutrition* 8:4.

17. Iwao et al. 1996. Effects of meal frequency on body composition during weight control in boxers. *Scandinavian Journal of Medicine and Science in Sports* 6(5): 265–72.

18. Arciero et al. 2013. Increased protein intake and meal frequency reduces abdominal fat during energy balance and energy deficit. *Obesity (Silver Spring)* 21(7): 1357–66.

19. Garrow et al. 1981. The effect of meal frequency and protein concentration on the composition of the weight lost by obese subjects. *British Journal of Nutrition* 45(1): 5–15.

20. Andersen et al. 1999. Effects of lifestyle activity vs structured aerobic exercise in obese women: A randomized trial. *JAMA: The Journal of the American Medical Association* 281(4): 335–40.

21. Feinman, R.D., and Fine, E.J. 2004. "A calorie is a calorie'" violates the second law of thermodynamics. *Nutrition Journal* 3:9.

22. Westerterp-Plantenga et al. 1999. Satiety related to 24 h diet-induced thermogenesis during high-protein/carbohydrate vs. high-fat diets measured in a respiration chamber. *European Journal of Clinical Nutrition* 53(6): 495–502.

23. Veldhorst et al. 2009. Gluconeogenesis and energy expenditure after a high-protein, carbohydrate-free diet. *American Journal of Clinical Nutrition* 90(3): 519–26.

24. Johnston et al. 2002. Postprandial thermogenesis is increased 100% on a high-protein, low-fat diet versus a high-carbohydrate, low-fat diet in healthy young women. *Journal of the American College of Nutrition* 21(1): 55–61.

25. Leidy et al. 2011. The effects of consuming frequent, higher-protein meals on appetite and satiety during weight loss in overweight/obese men. *Obesity (Silver Spring)* 19(4): 818–24.

26. Holt et al. 1995. A satiety index of common foods. *European Journal of Clinical Nutrition* 49(9): 675–90.

27. Devkota, S., and Layman, D.K. 2010. Protein metabolic roles in treatment of obesity. *Current Opinion in Clinical Nutrition and Metabolic Care* 13(4): 403–7.

28. Skov et al. 1999. Randomized trial on protein versus carbohydrate in ad libitum fat-reduced diet for the treatment of obesity. *International Journal of Obesity and Related Metabolic Disorders* 23(5): 528–36.

29. Parker et al. 2002. Effect of a high protein, high monounsaturated fat weight loss diet on glycemic control and lipid levels in type 2 diabetes. *Diabetes Care* 25(3): 425–30.

30. Foster et al. 2003. A randomized trial of a low carbohydrate diet for obesity. *New England Journal of Medicine* 348(21): 2082–90.

31. Mojtahedi et al. 2011. The effects of a higher protein intake during energy restriction on changes in body composition and physical function in older women. *Journals of Gerontology, Series A, Biological Sciences and Medical Sciences* 66(11): 1218–25.

32. Bopp et al. 2008. Lean mass loss is associated with low protein intake during dietary-induced weight loss in postmenopausal women. *Journal of the American Dietetic Association* 108(7): 1216–20.

33. Layman et al. 2003. A reduced ratio of dietary carbohydrate to protein improves body composition and blood lipid profiles during weight loss in adult women. *Journal of Nutrition* 133(2): 411–17.

34. Farnsworth et al. 2003. Effect of a high-protein, energy-restricted diet on body composition, glycemic control, and lipid concentrations in overweight and obese hyperinsulinemic men and women. *American Journal of Clinical Nutrition* 78(1): 31–39.

35. Layman et al. 2005. Dietary protein and exercise have additive effects on body composition during weight loss in adult women. *Journal of Nutrition* 135(8): 1903–10.

36. Skov et al. 1999. Randomized trial on protein versus carbohydrate in ad libitum fat-reduced diet for the treatment of obesity. *International Journal of Obesity and Related Metabolic Disorders* 23(5): 528–36.

37. Parker et al. 2002. Effect of a high-protein, high–monounsaturated fat weight-loss diet on glycemic control and lipid levels in type 2 diabetes. *Diabetes Care* 25(3): 425–30.

38. Leidy et al. 2011. Neural responses to visual food stimuli after a normal vs higher protein breakfast in breakfast-skipping teens: A pilot fMRI study. *Obesity (Silver Spring)* 19(10): 2019–25.

39. Paddon-Jones, D., and Leidy, H. 2014. Dietary protein and muscle in older persons. *Current Opinion in Clinical Nutrition and Metabolic Care* 17(1): 5–11.

40. FDA. Report on the Food and Drug Administration's review of the safety of recombinant bovine somatotropin. http://www.fda.gov/animalveterinary/safety-health/productsafetyinformation/ucm130321.htm. Accessed 4/29/14.

41. Wiley, A.S. 2011. Milk intake and total dairy consumption: Associations with early menarche in NHANES 1999–2004. *PLoS ONE* 6(2): e14685.

42. Leidy et al. 2009. Increased dietary protein consumed at breakfast leads to an initial and sustained feeling of fullness during energy restriction compared to other mealtimes. *British Journal of Nutrition* 101(6): 798–803.

43. Leidy et al. 2013. Beneficial effects of a higher-protein breakfast on the appetitive, hormonal, and neural signals controlling energy intake regulation in overweight/obese, "breakfast-skipping," late-adolescent girls. *American Journal of Clinical Nutrition* 97(4): 677–88.

44. Bayham et al. 2014. A randomized trial to manipulate the quality instead of quantity of dietary proteins to influence the markers of satiety. *Journal of Diabetes and Its Complications* 13. pii: S1056-8727 (14)00044-0.

45. Keogh, J.B., and Clifton, P. 2008. The effect of meal replacements high in glycomacropeptide on weight loss and markers of cardiovascular disease risk. *American Journal of Clinical Nutrition* 87(6): 1602–5.

46. Merchant et al. 2009. Carbohydrate intake and overweight and obesity among healthy adults. *Journal of the American Dietetic Association* 109(7): 1165–72.

47. Jakicic et al. 2001. American College of Sports Medicine position stand: Appropriate intervention strategies for weight loss and prevention of weight regain for adults. *Medicine and Science in Sports and Exercise* 33(12): 2145–56.

48. Klem et al. 1997. A descriptive study of individuals successful at long-term maintenance of substantial weight loss. *American Journal of Clinical Nutrition* 66(2): 239–46.

49. Kimmons et al. 2009. Fruit and vegetable intake among adolescents and adults in the United States: Percentage meeting individualized recommendations. *Medscape Journal of Medicine* 11(1): 26.

50. Oyebode et al. 2014. Fruit and vegetable consumption and all-cause, cancer and CVD mortality: Analysis of Health Survey for England data. *Journal of Epidemiology and Community Health* 31.

51. Gärtner et al. 1997. Lycopene is more bioavailable from tomato paste than from fresh tomatoes. *American Journal of Clinical Nutrition* 66(1): 116–22.

52. Anderson et al. 2009. Health benefits of dietary fiber. *Nutrition Reviews* 67(4): 188–205.

53. Bazzano et al. 2003. Dietary fiber intake and reduced risk of coronary heart disease in US men and women: The National Health and Nutrition Examination Survey I Epidemiologic Follow-Up Study. *Archives of Internal Medicine* 163(16): 1897–904.

54. Aune et al. 2011. Dietary fibre, whole grains, and risk of colorectal cancer: Systematic review and dose–response meta-analysis of prospective studies. *British Medical Journal* 343:d6617.

55. Threapleton et al. 2013. Dietary fiber intake and risk of first stroke: A systematic review and meta-analysis. *Stroke* 44(5): 1360–68.

56. Howarth et al. 2005. Dietary fiber and fat are associated with excess weight in young and middle-aged US adults. *Journal of the American Dietetic Association* 105(9): 1365–72.

57. Howarth et al. 2001. Dietary fiber and weight regulation. *Nutrition Reviews* 59(5): 129–39.

58. Buckley, J.D., and Howe, P.R. 2010. Long-chain omega-3 polyunsaturated fatty acids may be beneficial for obesity—a review. *Nutrients* 2(12): 1212–30.

59. Mattes, R.D. 2008. The energetics of nut consumption. *Asia Pacific Journal of Clinical Nutrition* 17(Suppl 1): 337–39.

60. Dreher, M.L., and Davenport, A.J. 2013. Hass avocado composition and potential health effects. *Critical Reviews in Food Science and Nutrition* 53(7): 738–50.

61. Buckley, J.D., and Howe, P.R. 2010. Long-chain omega-3 polyunsaturated fatty acids may be beneficial for obesity—a review. *Nutrients* 2(12): 1212–30.

62. Brufau et al. 2006. Nuts: Source of energy and macronutrients. *British Journal of Nutrition* 96 (Suppl 2): S24–28.

63. Harvard School of Public Health. 2014. Omega-3 fatty acids: An essential contribution. *Nutrition Source.* http://www.hsph.harvard.edu/nutritionsource/omega-3-fats. Accessed 4/29/14.

64. Li et al. 2013. Hass avocado modulates postprandial vascular reactivity and postprandial inflammatory responses to a hamburger meal in healthy volunteers. *Food and Function* 4(3): 384–91.

65. Foster et al. 2012. A randomized trial of the effects of an almond-enriched, hypocaloric diet in the treatment of obesity. *American Journal of Clinical Nutrition* 96(2): 249–54.

66. Schieberle et al. 2009–12. Identifying substances that regulate satiety in oils and fats and improving low-fat foodstuffs by adding lipid compounds with a high satiety effect; key findings of the DFG/AiF cluster project "Perception of fat content and regulating satiety: An approach to developing low-fat foodstuffs." *Technische Universitaet Muenchen.*

67. Rajaram et al. 2009. Walnuts and fatty fish influence different serum lipid fractions in normal to mildly hyperlipidemic individuals: A randomized controlled study. *American Journal of Clinical Nutrition* 89(5): 1657S–63S.

CHAPTER 2: FLEX YOUR MUSCLES DAILY

1. Hass et al. 2000. Single versus multiple sets in long-term recreational weightlifters. *Medicine and Science in Sports and Exercise* 32(1): 235–42.

2. Paoli et al. 2012. High-Intensity Interval Resistance Training (HIRT) influences resting energy expenditure and respiratory ratio in non-dieting individuals. *Journal of Translational Medicine* 10: 237.

3. Raynor et al. 2014. Physical activity variety, energy expenditure, and body mass index. *American Journal of Health Behavior* 38(4): 624–30.

4. Franklin, B.A. Program factors that influence exercise adherence: Practical adherence for the clinical staff. In Dishman, R.K., ed. 1988. Exercise adherence: Its impact on public health. Champaign, IL: Human Kinetics; 237–258.

5. Physical Activity Guidelines Advisory Committee. 2008. Physical Activity Guidelines Advisory Committee Report, 2008. Washington, DC: U.S. Department of Health and Human Services; 683.

6. Pedersen et al. 1999. Exercise and the immune system: Influence of nutrition and ageing. *Journal of Science and Medicine in Sport* 2(3): 234–52.

7. Jeurissen et al. 2003. The effects of physical exercise on the immune system. *Nederlands Tijdschrift Voor Geneeskunde* 147(28): 1347–51.

8. Pedersen, B.K., and Toft, A.D. 2000. Effects of exercise on lymphocytes and cytokines. *British Journal of Sports Medicine* 34(4): 246–51.

9. Gleeson, M. 2007. Immune function in sport and exercise. *Journal of Applied Physiology* 103(2): 693–99.

10. Baker et al. 2013. Strength and body composition changes in recreationally strength-trained individuals: Comparison of one versus three sets resistance-training programmes. *BioMed Research International* 615901.

11. Hass et al. 2000. Single versus multiple sets in long-term recreational weightlifters. *Medicine and Science in Sports and Exercise* 32(1): 235–42.

12. Heden et al. 2011. One-set resistance training elevates energy expenditure for 72 h similar to three sets. *European Journal of Applied Physiology* 111(3): 477–84.

13. Paoli et al. 2012. High-Intensity Interval Resistance Training (HIRT) influences resting energy expenditure and respiratory ratio in non-dieting individuals. *Journal of Translational Medicine* 10: 237.

14. Kirk et al. 2009. Minimal resistance training improves daily energy expenditure and fat oxidation. *Medicine and Science in Sports and Exercise* 41(5): 1122–29.

15. Winett et al. 2009. Initiating and maintaining resistance training in older adults: A social cognitive theory-based approach. *British Journal of Sports Medicine* 43(2): 114–19.

16. Hurley, B.F., and Roth, S.M. 2000. Strength training in the elderly: Effects on risk factors for age-related diseases. *Sports Medicine* 30(4): 249–68.

17. Winett, R.A., and Carpinelli, R.N. 2001. Potential health-related benefits of resistance training. *Preventive Medicine* 33(5): 503–13.

18. Hurley, B.F., and Roth, S.M. 2000. Strength training in the elderly: Effects on risk factors for age-related diseases. *Sports Medicine* 30(4): 249–68.

19. Francois et al. 2014. "Exercise snacks" before meals: A novel strategy to improve glycaemic control in individuals with insulin resistance. *Diabetologia* May 2014 [Epub ahead of print].

20. Campbell et al. 1994. Increased energy requirements and changes in body composition with resistance training in older adults. *American Journal of Clinical Nutrition* 60(2): 167–75.

21. Donnelly et al. 2009. Appropriate physical activity intervention strategies for weight loss and prevention of weight regain for adults. *Medicine and Science in Sports and Exercise* 41(2): 459–71.

22. Avila et al. 2010. Effect of moderate-intensity resistance training during weight loss on body composition and physical performance in overweight older adults. *European Journal of Applied Physiology* 109(3): 517–25.

23. Park et al. 2003. The effect of combined aerobic and resistance exercise training on abdominal fat in obese middle-aged women. *Journal of Physiological Anthropology and Applied Human Science* 22(3): 129–35.

24. Schoenfeld, B.J. 2013. Postexercise hypertrophic adaptations: A reexamination of the hormone hypothesis and its applicability to resistance training program design. *Journal of Strength and Conditioning Research* 27(6): 1720–30.

25. Mitchell et al. 2003. Resistance training prevents vertebral osteoporosis in lung transplant recipients. *Transplantation* 76(3): 557–62.

26. Winett, R.A., and Carpinelli, R.N. 2001. Potential health-related benefits of resistance training. *Preventive Medicine* 33(5): 503–13.

27. Williams, M.A., and Stewart, K.J. 2009. Impact of strength and resistance training on cardiovascular disease risk factors and outcomes in older adults. *Clinics in Geriatric Medicine* 25(4): 703–14.

28. Trudelle-Jackson et al. 2011. Relations of meeting national public health recommendations for muscular strengthening activities with strength, body composition, and obesity: The Women's Injury Study. *American Journal of Public Health* 101(10): 1930–35.

29. Botero et al. 2013. Effects of long-term periodized resistance training on body composition, leptin, resistin and muscle strength in elderly post-menopausal women. *Journal of Sports Medicine and Physical Fitness* 53(3): 289–94.

30. Pollock et al. 2000. American Heart Association Science Advisory. Resistance exercise in individuals with and without cardiovascular disease: Benefits, rationale, safety, and prescription—an advisory from the Committee on Exercise, Rehabilitation, and Prevention, Council on Clinical Cardiology, American Heart Association; position paper endorsed by the American College of Sports Medicine. *Circulation* 101(7): 828–33.

31. Schuenke et al. 2002. Effect of an acute period of resistance exercise on excess post-exercise oxygen consumption: Implications for body mass management. *European Journal of Applied Physiology* 86(5): 411–17.

32. Dionigi, R. 2007. Resistance training and older adults' beliefs about psychological benefits: The importance of self-efficacy and social interaction. *Journal of Sport and Exercise Psychology* 29(6): 723–46.

33. Latimer, A.E., and Ginis, K.A. 2005. Change in self-efficacy following a single strength-training session predicts sedentary older adults' subsequent motivation to join a strength-training program. *American Journal of Health Promotion* 20(2): 135–38.

34. Campbell et al. 1994. Increased energy requirements and changes in body composition with resistance training in older adults. *American Journal of Clinical Nutrition* 60: 167–75.

35. Pratley et al. 1994. Strength training increases resting metabolic rate and norepinephrine levels in healthy, 50- to 65-year-old men. *Journal of Applied Physiology* 76(1): 133–37.

36. Fell, James. The truth about boosting metabolism. http://www.chatelaine.com/health/fitness/the-truth-about-boosting-your-metabolism. Accessed 5/1/14.

37. Devlin et al. 1987. Enhanced peripheral and splanchic insulin sensitivity in NIDDM after single bout of exercise. *Diabetes* 36(4): 434–39.

38. Borghouts, L.B., and Keizer, H.A. 2000. Exercise and insulin sensitivity: A review. *International Journal of Sports Medicine* 21(1): 1–12.

39. Fiatarone et al. 1994. Exercise training and nutritional supplementation for physical frailty in very elderly people. *New England Journal of Medicine* 330(25): 1769–75.

40. Walker et al. 2000. Longitudinal evaluation of supervised versus unsupervised exercise programs for the treatment of osteoporosis. *European Journal of Applied Physiology* 83(4–5): 349–55.

41. Hurley, B.F., and Roth, S.M. 2000. Strength training in the elderly: Effects on risk factors for age-related diseases. *Sports Medicine* 30(4): 249–68.

42. Dela, F., and Kjaer, M. 2006. Resistance training, insulin sensitivity and muscle function in the elderly. *Essays in Biochemistry* 42: 75–88.

43. Guadalupe-Grau et al. 2009. Exercise and bone mass in adults. *Sports Medicine* 39(6): 439–68.

44. Nelson et al. 1994. Effects of high-intensity strength training on multiple risk factors for osteoporotic fractures: A randomized controlled trial. *JAMA: The Journal of the American Medical Association* 272(24): 1909–14.

45. Williams, M.A., and Stewart, K.J. 2009. Impact of strength and resistance training on cardiovascular disease risk factors and outcomes in older adults. *Clinics in Geriatric Medicine* 25(4): 703–14.

46. Donnelly et al. 2009. Appropriate physical activity intervention strategies for weight loss and prevention of weight regain for adults. *Medicine and Science in Sports and Exercise* 41(2): 459–71.

47. Kirk et al. 2009. Minimal resistance training improves daily energy expenditure and fat oxidation. *Medicine and Science in Sports and Exercise* 41(5): 1122–29.

48. Bea et al. 2010. Resistance training predicts 6-yr body composition change in postmenopausal women. *Medicine and Science in Sports and Exercise* 42(7): 1286–95.

CHAPTER 3: WALK IT OFF

1. Bassett et al. 2004. Physical activity in an Old Order Amish community. *Medicine and Science in Sports and Exercise* 36(1): 79–85.

2. Bassett et al. 2010. Pedometer-measured physical activity and health behaviors in U.S. adults. *Medicine and Science in Sports and Exercise* 42(10): 1819–25.

3. Eichholzer et al. 2005. Nutrition in Switzerland 2002: Results of the Swiss Health Survey. *Praxis* 94(44): 1713–21.

4. Yoshiike N., Kaneda F., and Takimoto, H. 2002. Epidemiology of obesity and public health strategies for its control in Japan. *Asia Pacific Journal of Clinical Nutrition* 11 (Suppl 8): S727–31.

5. Inoue, S., et al. 2006. Physical activity among the Japanese: Results of the National Health and Nutrition Survey. Proceedings of the International Congress on Physical Activity and Public Health; April 17–20; Atlanta, GA: U.S. Department of Health and Human Services; 79.

6. Sequeira et al. 1995. Physical activity assessment using a pedometer and its comparison with a questionnaire in a large population study. *American Journal of Epidemiology* 142(9): 989–99.

7. Tudor-Locke, C., and Bassett, D.R. Jr. 2004. How many steps/day are enough? Preliminary pedometer indices for public health. *Sports Medicine* 34(1): 1–8.

8. Donnelly et al. 2009. American College of Sports Medicine Position Stand. Appropriate physical activity intervention strategies for weight loss and prevention of weight regain for adults. *Medicine and Science in Sports and Exercise* 41(2): 459–71.

9. Jakicic et al. 2003. Effect of exercise duration and intensity on weight loss in overweight, sedentary women: A randomized trial. *JAMA: The Journal of the American Medical Association* 290(10): 1323–30.

10. Irwin et al. 2009. Exercise improves body fat, lean mass, and bone mass in breast cancer survivors. *Obesity (Silver Spring)* 7(8): 1534–41.

11. Manson et al. 2002. Walking compared with vigorous exercise for the prevention of cardiovascular events in women. *New England Journal of Medicine* 347(10): 716–25.

12. Thomas et al. 2012. The effects of aerobic activity on brain structure. *Frontiers in Psychology* 3: 86.

13. Murphy et al. 2002. Accumulating brisk walking for fitness, cardiovascular risk, and psychological health. *Medicine and Science in Sports and Exercise* 34(9): 1468–74.

14. Lee, M.R., and Kim, W.S. 2006. The effects of brisk walking versus brisk walking plus diet on triglycerides and apolipoprotein B levels in middle-aged overweight/obese women with high triglyceride levels. *Taehan Kanho Hakhoe Chi* 36(8): 1352–58.

15. Chien et al. 2000. Efficacy of a 24-week aerobic exercise program for osteopenic postmenopausal women. *Calcified Tissue International* 67(6): 443–48.

16. Walker et al. 2000. Longitudinal evaluation of supervised versus unsupervised exercise programs for the treatment of osteoporosis. *European Journal of Applied Physiology* 83(4–5): 349–55.

17. Hasbum et al. 2006. Effects of a controlled program of moderate physical exercise on insulin sensitivity in nonobese, nondiabetic subjects. *Clinical Journal of Sport Medicine* 16(1): 46–50.

18. Colberg et al. 2010. Exercise and type 2 diabetes: The American College of Sports Medicine and the American Diabetes Association—joint position statement. *Diabetes Care* 33(12): e147–67.

19. Moreau et al. 2001. Increasing daily walking lowers blood pressure in postmenopausal women. *Medicine and Science in Sports and Exercise* 33(11): 1825–31.

20. Tully et al. 2005. Brisk walking, fitness, and cardiovascular risk: A randomized controlled trial in primary care. *Preventive Medicine* 41(2): 622–28.

21. Murphy et al. 2002. Accumulating brisk walking for fitness, cardiovascular risk, and psychological health. *Medicine and Science in Sports and Exercise* 34(9): 1468–74.

22. Passos et al. 2010. Effect of acute physical exercise on patients with chronic primary insomnia. *Journal of Clinical Sleep Medicine* 6(3): 270–75.

23. Schoster et al. 2005. The People with Arthritis Can Exercise (PACE) program: A qualitative evaluation of participant satisfaction. *Preventing Chronic Disease* 2(3): A11.

24. Chubak et al. 2006. Moderate-intensity exercise reduces the incidence of colds among postmenopausal women. *American Journal of Medicine* 119(11): 937–42.

25. Martin et al. 2009. Exercise and respiratory tract viral infections. *Exercise and Sport Sciences Reviews* 37(4): 157–64.

26. Choi et al. 2007. Daily step goal of 10,000 steps: A literature review. *Clinical and Investigative Medicine* 30(3): E146–51.

27. Richardson et al. 2005. Feasibility of adding enhanced pedometer feedback to nutritional counseling for weight loss. *Journal of Medical Internet Research* 7(5): e56.

28. Hornbuckle, L.M., et al. 2005. Pedometer-determined walking and body composition variables in African-American women. *Medicine and Science in Sports and Exercise* 37(6): 1069–74.

29. Wyatt et al. 2005. A Colorado statewide survey of walking and its relation to excessive weight. *Medicine and Science in Sports and Exercise* 37(5): 724–30.

30. Tudor-Locke et al. 2004. Descriptive epidemiology of pedometer-determined physical activity. *Medicine and Science in Sports and Exercise* 36(9): 1567–73.

31. Krumm et al. 2006. The relationship between daily steps and body composition in postmenopausal women. *Journal of Women's Health* 15(2): 202–10.

32. Thompson et al. 2004. Relationship between accumulated walking and body composition in middle-aged women. *Medicine and Science in Sports and Exercise* 36(5): 911–14.

33. Levine, J.A. 2007. Nonexercise activity thermogenesis: Liberating the life force. *Journal of International Medicine* 262(3): 273–87.

34. Pescatello, L.S. 2001. Exercising for health the merits of lifestyle physical activity. *Western Journal of Medicine* 174(2): 114–18.

35. Haskell, W.L. 1994. Health consequences of physical activity: understanding and challenges regarding dose-response. *Medicine and Science in Sports and Exercise* 26(6): 649–60.

36. Damecour et al. 2010. Comparison of two heights for forward-placed trunk support with standing work. *Applied Ergonomics* 41(4): 536–41.

37. Reiff et al. 2012. Difference in caloric expenditure in sitting versus standing desks. *Journal of Physical Activity and Health* 9(7): 1009–11.

38. Levine, J.A., and Miller, J.M. 2007. The energy expenditure of using a "walk-and-work" desk for office workers with obesity. *British Journal of Sports Medicine* 41(9): 556–58.

39. Kobriger et al. 2006. The contribution of golf to daily physical activity recommendations: How many steps does it take to complete a round of golf? *Mayo Clinic Proceedings* 81(8): 1041–43.

40. Wing, R.R., and Jeffery, R.W. 1999. Benefits of recruiting participants with friends and increasing social support for weight loss and maintenance. *Journal of Consulting and Clinical Psychology* 67(1): 132–38.

41. Eberhardt, M.S., and Pamuk, E.R. 2004. The importance of place of residence: examining health in rural and nonrural areas. *American Journal of Public Health* 94(10): 1682–86.

42. Garden, F.L., and Jalaludin, B.B. 2009. Impact of urban sprawl on overweight, obesity, and physical activity in Sydney, Australia. *Journal of Urban Health* 86(1): 19–30.

43. Frank et al. 2004. Obesity relationships with community design, physical activity, and time spent in cars. *American Journal of Preventive Medicine* 27(2): 87–96.

44. Audrey et al. 2014. The contribution of walking to work to adult physical activity levels: A cross-sectional study. *International Journal of Behavioral Nutrition and Physical Activity* 11: 37.

45. Bassett et al. 2008. Walking, cycling, and obesity rates in Europe, North America, and Australia. *Journal of Physical Activity and Health* 5(6): 795–814.

46. Badland et al. 2010. How does car parking availability and public transport accessibility influence work-related travel behaviors? *Sustainability* 2(2): 576–90.

47. Lindstrom, M. 2008. Means of transportation to work and overweight and obesity: A population-based study in southern Sweden. *Preventive Medicine* 46(1): 22–28.

48. Bassett et al. 2010. Pedometer-measured physical activity and health behaviors in U.S. adults. *Medicine and Science in Sports and Exercise* 42(10): 1819–25.

49. Jakes et al. 2003. Television viewing and low participation in vigorous recreation are independently associated with obesity and markers of cardiovascular disease risk: EPIC-Norfolk population-based study. *European Journal of Clinical Nutrition* 57(9): 1089–96.

50. Stamatakis et al. 2009. Moderate-to-vigorous physical activity and sedentary behaviours in relation to body mass index–defined and waist circumference–defined obesity. *British Journal of Nutrition* 101(5): 765–73.

51. Healy et al. 2008. Objectively measured sedentary time, physical activity, and metabolic risk: The Australian Diabetes, Obesity and Lifestyle Study. *Diabetes Care* 31(2): 369–71.

52. Stamatakis, E., and Hamer, M. 2011. Sedentary behaviour: Redefining its meaning and links to chronic disease. *British Journal of Hospital Medicine* 72(4): 192–95.

53. Patel et al. 2010. Leisure time spent sitting in relation to total mortality in a prospective cohort of U.S. adults. *American Journal of Epidemiology* 172(4): 419–29.

54. Katzmarzyk et al. 2009. Sitting time and mortality from all causes, cardiovascular disease, and cancer. *Medicine and Science in Sports and Exercise* 41(5): 998–1005.

55. Friedenreich et al. 2010. State of the epidemiological evidence on physical activity and cancer prevention. *European Journal of Cancer* 46(14): 2593–604.

56. Veerman et al. 2012. Television viewing time and reduced life expectancy: A life table analysis. *British Journal of Sports Medicine* 46(13): 927–30.

57. de Jonge, L., et al. 2010. Impact of 6-month caloric restriction on autonomic nervous system activity in healthy, overweight, individuals. *Obesity (Silver Spring)* 18(2): 414–16.

58. Gordon-Larsen et al. 2009. Fifteen-year longitudinal trends in walking patterns and their impact on weight change. *American Journal of Clinical Nutrition* 89(1): 19–26.

59. Haskell et al. 2007. Physical activity and public health: Updated recommendation for adults from the American College of Sports Medicine and the American Heart Association. *Medicine and Science in Sports and Exercise* 39(8): 1423–34.

60. Focht, B. 2013. Affective responses to 10-minute and 30-minute walks in sedentary, overweight women: Relationships with theory-based correlates of walking for exercise. *Psychology of Sport and Exercise* 14(5): 759–66.

61. Williams, P.T., and Thompson, P.D. 2013. Walking versus running for hypertension, cholesterol, and diabetes mellitus risk reduction. *Arteriosclerosis, Thrombosis, and Vascular Biology* 33(5): 1085–91.

62. U.S. Department of Health and Human Services, Centers for Disease Control and Prevention. 1996. *Physical activity and health: A report of the Surgeon General.* Atlanta, GA: Centers for Disease Control and Prevention, National Center for Chronic Disease Prevention and Health Promotion, Division of Nutrition and Physical Activity. http://www.cdc.gov/nccdphp/sgr/sgr.htm.

63. Woodcock et al. 2011. Non-vigorous physical activity and all-cause mortality: Systematic review and meta-analysis of cohort studies. *International Journal of Epidemiology* 40(1): 121–38.

64. Church et al. 2009. Changes in weight, waist circumference and compensatory responses with different doses of exercise among sedentary, overweight postmenopausal women. *PLoS One* 4(2): e4515.

65. MacLean et al. 2006. Peripheral metabolic responses to prolonged weight reduction that promote rapid, efficient regain in obesity-prone rats. *American Journal of Physiology* 290(6): R1577–88.

66. Melanson et al. 2009. When energy balance is maintained, exercise does not induce negative fat balance in lean sedentary, obese sedentary, or lean endurance-trained individuals. *Journal of Applied Physiology* 107(6): 1847–56.

67. Hagobian et al. 2009. Effects of exercise on energy-regulating hormones and appetite in men and women. *American Journal of Physiology: Regulatory, Integrative and Comparative Physiology* 296(2): R233–42.

68. Murphy et al. 2008. Exercise stress increases susceptibility to influenza infection. *Brain, Behavior, and Immunity* 22(8): 1152–55.

69. Lowder et al. 2005. Moderate exercise protects mice from death due to influenza virus. *Brain, Behavior, and Immunity* 19(5): 377–80.

70. Suzuki et al. 2002. Systemic inflammatory response to exhaustive exercise. Cytokine kinetics. *Exercise Immunology Review* 8: 6–48.

71. Rosa et al. 2011. Exhaustive exercise increases inflammatory response via Toll like receptor-4 and NF-κBp65 pathway in rat adipose tissue. *Journal of Cellular Physiology* 226(6): 1604–7.

72. Rippe et al. 1998. Improved psychological well-being, quality of life, and health practices in moderately overweight women participating in a 12-week structured weight-loss program. *Obesity Research* 6(3): 208–18.

73. Passos et al. 2010. Effect of acute physical exercise on patients with chronic primary insomnia. *Journal of Clinical Sleep Medicine* 6(3): 270–75.

74. Hillman et al. 2009. Aerobic fitness and cognitive development: Event-related brain potential and task performance indices of executive control in preadolescent children. *Developmental Psychology* 45(1): 114–29.

75. Aberg et al. 2009. Cardiovascular fitness is associated with cognition in young adulthood. *Proceedings of the National Academy of Sciences of the United States of America* 106(49): 20906–11.

76. Oppezzo, M., and Schwartz, D.L. 2014. Give your ideas some legs: The positive effect of walking on creative thinking. *Journal of Experimental Psychology: Learning, Memory, and Cognition* [Epub ahead of print].

77. Nanda et al. 2013. The acute effects of a single bout of moderate-intensity aerobic exercise on cognitive functions in healthy adult males. *Journal of Clinical and Diagnostic Research* 7(9): 1883–85.

78. Schmidt-Kassow et al. 2013. Physical exercise during encoding improves vocabulary learning in young female adults: A neuroendocrinological study. *PLoS One* 8(5): e64172.

79. Stein, P.N., and Motta, R.W. 1992. Effects of aerobic and nonaerobic exercise on depression and self-concept. *Perceptual and Motor Skills* 74(1): 79 89.

80. Dimeo et al. 2001. Benefits from aerobic exercise in patients with major depression: A pilot study. *British Journal of Sports Medicine* 35(2): 114–17.

81. Hamer et al. 2009. A dose-response relationship between physical activity and mental health: The Scottish Health Survey. *British Journal of Sports Medicine* 43(14): 1111–14.

82. Yaffe et al. 2001. A prospective study of physical activity and cognitive decline in elderly women: Women who walk. *Archives of Internal Medicine* 61(14): 1703–8.

83. Hall et al. 2004. Energy expenditure of walking and running: Comparison with prediction equations. *Medicine and Science in Sports and Exercise* 36(12): 2128–34.

84. Adapted from Cameron et al. 2004. Energy expenditure of walking and running. *Medicine and Science in Sport and Exercise* 36(12): 2128–34.

85. Bravata et al. 2007. Using pedometers to increase physical activity and improve health. *JAMA: The Journal of the American Medical Association* 298(19): 2296–304.

86. Bravata et al. 2007. Using pedometers to increase physical activity and improve health. *JAMA: The Journal of the American Medical Association* 298(19): 2296–304.

87. Snyder et al. 2011. Pedometer use increases daily steps and functional status in older adults. *Journal of the American Medical Directors Association* 12(8): 590–94.

88. Richardson et al. 2008. A meta-analysis of pedometer-based walking interventions and weight loss. *Annals of Family Medicine* 6(1): 69–77.

89. Bravata et al. 2007. Using pedometers to increase physical activity and improve health. *JAMA: The Journal of the American Medical Association* 298(19): 2296–304.

90. Lee et al. 2010. Physical activity and weight-gain prevention. *JAMA: The Journal of the American Medical Association* 303(12): 1173–79.

CHAPTER 4: SNOOZE TO LOSE

1. Huffington, A. 2014. *Thrive: The Third Metric to Redefining Success and Creating a Life of Well-Being, Wisdom, and Wonder.* Harmony/Crown: New York.

2. Spiegel et al. 2004. Sleep curtailment in healthy young men is associated with decreased leptin levels, elevated ghrelin levels, and increased hunger and appetite. *Annals of Internal Medicine* 141(11): 846–850.

3. Kripke et al. 1979. Short and long sleep and sleeping pills: Is increased mortality associated? *Archives of General Psychiatry* 36(1): 103–16.

4. National Sleep Foundation. Sleep in America Poll, 2001–2002. Washington, DC.

5. Lerman et al. 2012. Fatigue risk management in the workplace. *Journal of Occupational and Environmental Medicine* 54(2): 231–58.

6. Harrison, E.M., and Gorman, M.R. 2012. Changing the waveform of circadian rhythms: Considerations for shift-work. *Frontiers in Neurology* 3: 72.

7. Spivey, A. 2010. Lose sleep, gain weight: Another piece of the obesity puzzle. *Environmental Health Perspectives* 118(1): A28–33.

8. Steptoe et al. 2008. Positive affect, psychological well-being, and good sleep. *Journal of Psychosomatic Research* 64(4): 409–15.

9. Roberts et al. 2000. Sleep complaints and depression in an aging cohort: A prospective perspective. *American Journal of Psychiatry* 157(1): 81–88.

10. Sekine et al. 2006. Work and family characteristics as determinants of socioeconomic and sex inequalities in sleep: The Japanese Civil Servants Study. *Sleep* 29(2): 206–16.

11. Akerstedt et al. 2002. Sleep disturbances, work stress and work hours: A cross-sectional study. *Journal of Psychosomatic Research* 53(3): 741–48.

12. Li, G., and Haslegrave, C.M. 1999. Seated postures for manual, visual and combined tasks. *Ergonomics* 42(8): 1060–86.

13. Alvarez, G.G., and Ayas, N.T. 2004. The impact of daily sleep duration on health: A review of the literature. *Progress in Cardiovascular Nursing* 19(2): 56–59.

14. Pires et al. 2012. Relationship between sleep deprivation and anxiety: Experimental research perspective. *Einstein* (São Paulo) 10(4): 519–23.

15. Wilder-Smith et al. 2013. Impact of partial sleep deprivation on immune markers. *Sleep Medicine* 14(10): 1031–34.

16. Knutson et al. 2007. The metabolic consequences of sleep deprivation. *Sleep Medicine Reviews* 11(3): 163–78.

17. Trenell et al. 2007. Sleep and metabolic control: Waking to a problem? *Clinical and Experimental Pharmacology and Physiology* 34(1–2): 1–9.

18. Gottlieb et al. 2005. Association of sleep time with diabetes mellitus and impaired glucose tolerance. *Archives of Internal Medicine* 165(8): 863–67.

19. Donga et al. 2010. A single night of partial sleep deprivation induces insulin resistance in multiple metabolic pathways in healthy subjects. *Journal of Clinical Endocrinology and Metabolism* 95(6): 2963–68.

20. Buxton et al. 2010. Sleep restriction for 1 week reduces insulin sensitivity in healthy men. *Diabetes* 59(9): 2126–33.

21. Spiegel et al. 2005. Sleep loss: A novel risk factor for insulin resistance and type 2 diabetes. *Journal of Applied Physiology* 99(5): 2008–19.

22. Leproult, R., and Van Cauter, E. 2010. Role of sleep and sleep loss in hormonal release and metabolism. *Endocrine Development* 17: 11–21.

23. Ayas et al. 2003. A prospective study of self-reported sleep duration and incident diabetes in women. *Diabetes Care* 26(2): 380–84.

24. Chaput et al. 2014. Change in sleep duration and visceral fat accumulation over 6 years in adults. *Obesity* 22(5): E9–12.

25. Gangwisch et al. 2005. Inadequate sleep as a risk factor for obesity: Analyses of the NHANES I. *Sleep* 28(10): 1289–96.

26. Hasler et al. 2004. The association between short sleep duration and obesity in young adults: A 13-year prospective study. *Sleep* 27(4): 661–66.

27. Watson et al. 2010. A twin study of sleep duration and body mass index. *Journal of Clinical Sleep Medicine* 6(1): 11–17.

28. Nutt et al. 2008. Sleep disorders as core symptoms of depression. *Dialogues in Clinical Neuroscience* 10(3): 329–36.

29. Jindal, R.D., and Thase, M.E. 2004. Treatment of insomnia associated with clinical depression. *Sleep Medicine Reviews* 8(1): 19–30.

30. Franzen, P.L., and Buysse, D.J. 2008. Sleep disturbances and depression: Risk relationships for subsequent depression and therapeutic implications. *Dialogues in Clinical Neuroscience* 10(4): 473–81.

31. Taheri et al. 2004. Short sleep duration is associated with reduced leptin, elevated ghrelin, and increased body mass index. *PLoS Medicine* 1(3): e62.

32. Spiegel et al. 2004. Sleep curtailment in healthy young men is associated with decreased leptin levels, elevated ghrelin levels, and increased hunger and appetite. *Annals of Internal Medicine* 141(11): 846–50.

33. Taheri et al. 2004. Short sleep duration is associated with reduced leptin, elevated ghrelin, and increased body mass index. *PLoS Medicine* 1(3): e62.

34. Reid et al. 2014. Timing and intensity of light correlate with body weight in adults. *PLoS One* 9(4): e92251.

35. Spiegel et al. 1999. Impact of sleep debt on metabolic and endocrine function. *Lancet* 354(9188): 1435–39.

36. Leproult et al. 1997. Sleep loss results in an elevation of cortisol levels the next evening. *Sleep* 20(10): 865–70.

37. Spiegel et al. 1999. Impact of sleep debt on metabolic and endocrine function. *Lancet* 354(9188): 1435–39.

38. Peuhkuri et al. 2012. Diet promotes sleep duration and quality. *Nutrition Research* 32(5): 309–19.

39. Peuhkuri et al. 2012. Diet promotes sleep duration and quality. *Nutrition Research* 32(5): 309–19.

40. Lande, R.G., and Gragnani, C. 2010. Nonpharmacologic approaches to the management of insomnia. *Journal of the American Osteopathic Association* 110(12): 695–01.

41. Reid et al. 2014. Timing and intensity of light correlate with body weight in adults. *PLoS One* 9(4): e92251.

42. Stevens et al. 2013. Adverse health effects of nighttime lighting: Comments on American Medical Association policy statement. *American Journal of Preventive Medicine* 45(3): 343–46.

43. Scheer et al. 2009. Adverse metabolic and cardiovascular consequences of circadian misalignment. *Proceedings of the National Academy of Sciences of the United States of America* 106(11): 4453–58.

44. Gooley et al. 2011. Exposure to room light before bedtime suppresses melatonin onset and shortens melatonin duration in humans. *Journal of Clinical Endocrinology and Metabolism* 96(3): E463–72.

45. Lockley et al. 2003. High sensitivity of the human circadian melatonin rhythm to resetting by short wavelength light. *Journal of Clinical Endocrinology and Metabolism* 88(9): 4502–5.

46. Holzman, D.C. 2010. What's in a color? The unique human health effects of blue light. *Environmental Health Perspectives* 118(1): A22–A27.

47. Greer et al. 2013. The impact of sleep deprivation on food desire in the human brain. *Nature Communications* 4: 2259.

48. Markwald et al. 2013. Impact of insufficient sleep on total daily energy expenditure, food intake, and weight gain. *Proceedings of the National Academy of Sciences of the United States of America* 110(14): 5695–700.

49. Chaput et al. 2011.The association between short sleep duration and weight gain is dependent on disinhibited eating behavior in adults. *Sleep* 34(10): 1291–97.

50. Chen et al. 2009. Sleep quality, depression state, and health status of older adults after silver yoga exercises: Cluster randomized trial. *International Journal of Nursing Studies* 46(2): 154–63.

51. Manjunath, N.K., and Telles, S. 2005. Influence of yoga and Ayurveda on self-rated sleep in a geriatric population. *Indian Journal of Medical Research* 121(5): 683–90.

52. Leopoldino et al. 2013. Effect of Pilates on sleep quality and quality of life of sedentary population. *Journal of Bodywork and Movement Therapies* 17(1): 5–10.

53. Caldwell et al. 2010. Developing mindfulness in college students through movement-based courses: Effects on self-regulatory self-efficacy, mood, stress, and sleep quality. *Journal of American College Health* 58(5): 433–42.

54. Caldwell et al. 2009. Effect of Pilates and aiji quan training on self-efficacy, sleep quality, mood, and physical performance of college students. *Journal of Bodywork and Movement Therapies* 13(2): 155–63.

55. Siqueira et al. 2010. Pilates method in personal autonomy, static balance and quality of life of elderly females. *Journal of Bodywork and Movement Therapies* 14(2): 195–202.

56. Chang et al. 2012. The effects of music on the sleep quality of adults with chronic insomnia using evidence from polysomnographic and self-reported analysis: A randomized control trial. *International Journal of Nursing Studies* 49(8): 921–30.

57. Harsora, P., and Kessman, J. 2009. Nonpharmacologic management of chronic insomnia. *American Family Physician* 79(2): 125–30.

58. Morin et al. 1999. Nonpharmacologic treatment of chronic insomnia. An American Academy of Sleep Medicine review. *Sleep* 22(8): 1134–56.

59. Richardson et al. 2007. Earplugs and eye masks: Do they improve critical care patients' sleep? *Nursing in Critical Care* 12(60): 278–86.

60. Hu et al. 2010. Effects of earplugs and eye masks on nocturnal sleep, melatonin and cortisol in a simulated intensive care unit environment. *Critical Care* 14(2): R66.

61. Xie et al. 2009. Clinical review: The impact of noise on patients' sleep and the effectiveness of noise reduction strategies in intensive care units. *Critical Care* 13(2): 208.

62. Wallace et al. 1999. The effect of earplugs on sleep measures during exposure to simulated intensive care unit noise. *American Journal of Critical Care* 8(4): 210–19.

63. Richardson et al. 2007. Earplugs and eye masks: Do they improve critical care patients' sleep? *Nursing in Critical Care* 12(60): 278–86.

64. Hu et al. 2010. Effects of earplugs and eye masks on nocturnal sleep, melatonin and cortisol in a simulated intensive care unit environment. *Critical Care* 14(2): R66.

65. Xie et al. 2009. Clinical review: The impact of noise on patients' sleep and the effectiveness of noise reduction strategies in intensive care units. *Critical Care* 13(2): 208.

66. Williamson, J.W. 1992. The effects of ocean sounds on sleep after coronary artery bypass graft surgery. *American Journal of Critical Care* 1(1): 91–97.

67. Stanchina et al. 2005. The influence of white noise on sleep in subjects exposed to ICU noise. *Sleep Medicine* 6(5): 423–28.

68. Kelly et al. 2012. Recent developments in home sleep-monitoring devices. *ISRN Neurology* 768794.

69. Sivertsen et al. 2009. Sleep and sleep disorders in chronic users of zopiclone and drug-free insomniacs. *Journal of Clinical Sleep Medicine* 5(4): 349–54.

70. Saul, S. October 23, 2007. Sleep drugs found only mildly effective, but wildly popular. *New York Times.*

71. Buscemi et al. 2007. The efficacy and safety of drug treatments for chronic insomnia in adults: A meta-analysis of RCTs. *Journal of General Internal Medicine* 22(9): 1335–50.

72. Inagaki, T., et al. 2010. Adverse reactions to zolpidem: Case reports and a review of the literature. *Primary Care Companion to the Journal of Clinical Psychiatry* 12(6): PCC.09r00849.

73. Jacobson et al. 2010. Effect of prescribed sleep surfaces on back pain and sleep quality in patients diagnosed with low back and shoulder pain. *Applied Ergonomics* 42(1): 91–97.

74. Addison et al. 1986. A survey of the United States public concerning the quality of sleep. *Sleep Research* 16: 244.

75. Jacobson et al. 2009. Changes in back pain, sleep quality, and perceived stress after introduction of new bedding systems. *Journal of Chiropractic Medicine* 8(1): 1–8.

76. Reinberg, S. Prescription sleep aids a common choice for American insomnia. HealthDay. http://consumer.healthday.com/sleep-disorder-information-33/misc-sleep-problems-news-626/prescription-sleep-aids-a-common-choice-for-american-insomnia-679670.html. Accessed 6/14/14.

77. Deschenes, C.L., and McCurry, S.M. 2009. Current treatments for sleep disturbances in individuals with dementia. *Current Psychiatry Reports* 11(1): 20–26.

78. Harsora P., and Kessman, J. 2009. Nonpharmacologic management of chronic insomnia. *American Family Physician* 79(2): 125–30.

79. Pallesen et al. 2003. Behavioral treatment of insomnia in older adults: An open clinical trial comparing two interventions. *Behaviour Research and Therapy* 41(1): 31–48.

80. Bootzin, R.R., and Rider, S.P. 1997. Behavioral techniques and biofeedback for insomnia. In Pressman, M.R., and Orr, W.C. (Eds.), *Understanding Sleep: The Evaluation and Treatment of Sleep Disorders.* Washington, DC: American Psychological Association; 315–38.

81. Lack et al. 1995. The treatment of sleep onset insomnia with morning bright light. *Sleep Research* 24A: 338.

82. King et al. 1997. Moderate-intensity exercise and self-rated quality of sleep in older adults: A randomized controlled trial. JAMA: *The Journal of the American Medical Association* 277(1): 32–37.

83. Troxel et al. 2010. Does social support differentially affect sleep in older adults with versus without insomnia? *Journal of Psychosomatic Research* 69(5): 459–66.

84. Ryff et al. 2004. Positive health: Connecting well-being with biology *Philosophical Transactions of the Royal Society Biological Sciences* 359(1449): 1383–94.

85. Tugade et al. 2004. Psychological resilience and positive emotional granularity: Examining the benefits of positive emotions on coping and health. *Journal of Personality* 72(6): 1161–90.

86. Emmons, R.A., and McCullough, M.E. 2003. Counting blessings versus burdens: An experimental investigation of gratitude and subjective well-being in daily life. *Journal of Personality and Social Psychology* 84(2): 377–89.

CHAPTER 5: PULL THE CORD

1. Nielsen Company. December 2013. A look across media: The cross platform report.

2. Lear, S.A., et al. 2014. The association between ownership of common household devices and obesity and diabetes in high, middle and low income countries. *Canadian Medical Association Journal* 186(4): 258–66.

3. Basner, M., and Dinges, DF. Dubious bargain: Trading sleep for Leno and Letterman. *Sleep* 32(6): 747–52.

4. Ogden, J., et al. 2013. Distraction: The desire to eat and food intake—towards an expanded model of mindless eating. *Appetite* 62: 119–26.

5. Bellissimo, N., et al. 2007. Effect of television viewing at mealtime on food intake after a glucose preload in boys. *Pediatric Research* 61(6): 745–49.

6. Temple, J.L., et al. 2007. Television watching increases motivated responding for food and energy intake in children. *American Journal of Clinical Nutrition* 85(2): 355–61.

7. Higgs, S., and Woodward, M. 2009. Television watching during lunch increases afternoon snack intake of young women. *Appetite* 52(1): 39–43.

8. Moray, J., et al. 2007. Viewing television while eating impairs the ability to accurately estimate total amount of food consumed. *Bariatric Nursing and Surgical Patient Care* 2: 71–76.

9. Wansink, B. 2010. From mindless eating to mindlessly eating better. *Physiology and Behavior* 100(5): 454–63.

10. Boulos et al. 2012. ObesiTV: How television is influencing the obesity epidemic. *Physiology and Behavior* 107(1): 146-53.

11. Blass et al. 2006. On the road to obesity: Television viewing increases intake of high-density foods. *Physiology and Behavior* 88(4–5): 597–604.

12. Liang et al. 2009. Nutrition and body weights of Canadian children watching television and eating while watching television. *Public Health Nutrition* 12(12): 2457–63.

13. Mittal et al. 2011. Snacking while watching TV impairs food recall and promotes food intake on a later TV free test meal. *Applied Cognitive Psychology* 25: 871–77.

14. Nielsen Company. December 2013. A look across media: The cross platform report.

15. Moray et al. 2007. Viewing television while eating impairs the ability to accurately estimate total amount of food consumed. *Bariatric Nursing and Surgical Patient Care* 2: 71–76.

16. Robinson, E., et al. 2013. Eating attentively: A systematic review and meta-analysis of the effect of food intake memory and awareness on eating. *American Journal of Clinical Nutrition* 97(4): 728–42.

17. Thorp et al. 2011. Sedentary behaviors and subsequent health outcomes in adults a systematic review of longitudinal studies, 1996–2011. *American Journal of Preventative Medicine* 41: 207–15.

18. Boulos et al. 2012. ObesiTV: How television is influencing the obesity epidemic. *Physiology and Behavior* 107(1): 146–53.

19. Otten et al. 2009. Effects of television viewing reduction on energy intake and expenditure in overweight and obese adults: A randomized controlled trial. *Archives of Internal Medicine* 169: 2109–15.

20. Shields, M., and Tremblay, M.S. 2008. Sedentary behaviour and obesity. *Health Reports* 19(2): 19–30.

21. Sugiyama et al. 2008. Is television viewing time a marker of a broader pattern of sedentary behavior? *Annals of Behavioral Medicine* 35(2): 245–50.

22. Deloitte. March 26, 2014. Digital omnivores craving more content across devices, according to Deloitte's "Digital Democracy Survey." http://www.deloitte.com/view/en_US/us/press/Press-Releases/483bcdcb4bfd4410VgnVCM3000003456f70aRCRD.htm.

23. Accenture. 2013. Video-over-Internet consumer survey. http://www.accenture.com/SiteCollection Documents/PDF/Accenture-Video-Over-Internet-Consumer-Survey-2013.pdf. Accessed 4/1/14.

24. Hu et al. 2003. Television watching and other sedentary behaviors in relation to risk of obesity and type 2 diabetes mellitus in women. *JAMA: The Journal of the American Medical Association* 289(14): 1785   91.

25. Katzmarzyk, P.T., and Lee, I.M. 2012. Sedentary behaviour and life expectancy in the USA: A cause-deleted life table analysis. *British Medical Journal Open* 2(4).

26. Owen et al. 2010. Too much sitting: The population-health science of sedentary behavior. *Exercise and Sport Sciences Reviews* 38(3): 105.

27. Nakazawa et al. 2002. Association between duration of daily VDT use and subjective symptoms. *American Journal of Industrial Medicine* 42(5): 421–26.

28. Sivaraman et al. 2011. Occupation related health hazards online survey among software engineers of south India. *Indian Journal of Medical Specialties* 2(1): 77–78.

29. Kesavachandran et al. 2006. Working conditions and health among employees at information technology–enabled services: A review of current evidence. *Indian Journal of Medical Science* 60: 300–307.

30. Talwar et al. 2009. A study of visual and musculoskeletal health disorders among computer professionals in NCR Delhi. *Indian Journal Community Medicine* 34: 326–28.

31. Suparna et al. 2005. Occupational health problems and role of ergonomics in information technology professionals in national capital region. *Indian Journal of Occupational and Environmental Medicine* 9(3): 111–14.

32. Chatterjee, A., and DeVol, R.C. 2012. Waistlines of the world: The effect of information and communications on obesity. Milken Institute. http://www.milkeninstitute.org/pdf/Waistlines-of-the-World.pdf. Accessed 5/3/14.

33. Vandelanotte et al. 2009. Associations of leisure-time Internet and computer use with overweight and obesity, physical activity and sedentary behaviors: Cross-sectional study. *Journal of Medical Internet Research* 11(3): e28.

34. Kohlhepp, J. 2014. Princeton: Huffington discusses book at university. *Princeton Packet*. http://www.centraljerseymarketplace.com/newsite/pp/story.cgi?section=news&story=doc53597ddd189e3808679628&s=1+page_1. Accessed 5/3/14.

35. Kross et al. 2013. Facebook use predicts declines in subjective well-being in young adults. *PLoS One* 8(8): e69841.

36. Ellison et al. 2007. The benefits of Facebook "friends": Social capital and college students' use of online social network sites. *Journal of Computer-Mediated Communication* 12(4): 1143–68.

37. Cotten et al. 2012. Internet use and depression among older adults. *Computers in Human Behavior* 28(2): 496–99.

38. Accenture. 2013. Video-over-Internet consumer survey. http://www.accenture.com /SiteCollection Documents/PDF/Accenture-Video-Over-Internet-Consumer-Survey-2013.pdf. Accessed 4/1/14.

39. Becker et al. 2013. Media multitasking is associated with symptoms of depression and social anxiety. *Cyberpsychology, Behavior Social Networking* 16(2): 132–35.

40. Boone et al. 2007. Screen time and physical activity during adolescence: Longitudinal effects on obesity in young adulthood. *International Journal of Behavioral Nutrition and Physical Activity* 4:26.

41. Henderson, V.R. 2007. Longitudinal associations between television viewing and body mass index among white and black girls. *Journal of Adolescent Health* 41: 544–50.

42. O'Brien et al. 2007. The ecology of childhood overweight: A 12-year longitudinal analysis. *International Journal of Obesity* 31: 1469–78.

43. Danner, F.W. 2008. A national longitudinal study of the association between hours of TV viewing and the trajectory of BMI growth among US children. *Journal of Pediatric Psychology* 33(10): 1100–107.

44. Robinson, T.N. 1999. Reducing children's television viewing to prevent obesity: A randomized controlled trial. *JAMA : The Journal of the American Medical Association* 282(16): 1561–567.

45. Landhuis et al. 2008. Programming obesity and poor fitness: The long-term impact of childhood television. *Obesity (Silver Spring)* 16(6): 1457–59.

46. Parsons et al. 2008. Television viewing and obesity: A prospective study in the 1958 British birth cohort. *European Journal of Clinical Nutrition* 62(12): 1355–63.

47. Garmy et al. 2012. Sleep and television and computer habits of Swedish school-age children. *Journal of School Nursing* 28(6): 469–76.

48. Shin, N. 2004. Exploring pathways from television viewing to academic achievement in school-age children. *Journal of Genetic Psychology* 165(4): 367–81.

49. Swing et al. 2010. Television and video game exposure and the development of attention problems. *Pediatrics* 126(2): 214–21.

50. Temple et al. 2007. Television watching increases motivated responding for food and energy intake in children. *American Journal of Clinical Nutrition* 85(2): 355–61.

51. Sonneville, K.R., and Gortmaker, S.L. 2008. Total energy intake, adolescent discretionary behaviors and the energy gap. *International Journal of Obesity* 32(Suppl 6): S19–27.

52. Miller et al. 2008. Association between television viewing and poor diet quality in young children. *International Journal of Pediatric Obesity* 3(3): 168–76.

53. Wiecha et al. 2008. When children eat what they watch: Impact of television viewing on dietary intake in youth. *Archives of Pediatrics and Adolescent Medicine* 160(4): 436–42.

54. Barr-Anderson, D.J., et al. 2009. Does television viewing predict dietary intake five years later in high school students and young adults? *International Journal of Behavior Nutrition and Physical Activity* 6:7.

55. Gentile, D. A., and Walsh, D. A. 2002. A normative study of family media habits. *Journal of Applied Developmental Psychology* 23: 157-178.

56. Gentile et al. 2014. Protective effects of parental monitoring of children's media use: A prospective study. *Journal of the American Medical Association Pediatrics* 168(5): 479–84.

57. Divan et al. 2012. Cellphone use and behavioural problems in young children. *Journal of Epidemiology and Community Health* 66(6): 524–29.

58. Gentile et al. 2014. Mediators and moderators of long-term effects of violent video games on aggressive behavior: Practice, thinking, and action. *Journal of the American Medical Association Pediatrics* 168(5): 450–57.

59. Maddison et al. 2011. Effects of active video games on body composition: A randomized controlled trial. *American Journal of Clinical Nutrition* 94(1): 156-63.

60. Figueiro et al. 2011. The impact of light from computer monitors on melatonin levels in college students. *Neuroendocrinology Letters* 32(2): 158–63.

61. Chellappa et al. 2012. Human melatonin and alerting response to blue-enriched light depend on a polymorphism in the clock gene PER3. *Journal of Clinical Endocrinology and Metabolism* 97(3): E433–37.

62. Wood et al. 2013. Light level and duration of exposure determine the impact of self-luminous tablets on melatonin suppression. *Applied Ergonomics* 44(2): 237–40.

63. Burkhart, K., and Phelps, J.R. 2009. Amber lenses to block blue light and improve sleep: A randomized trial. *Chronobiology International* 26(8): 1602–12.

64. Lily, P. 2014. AT&T and Verizon want to cut the POTS cord: Say goodbye to the landline http://global.ofweek.com/news/ AT-T-and-Verizon-want-to-cut-the-POTS-cord-Say-goodbye-to-the-landline-10071. Accessed 5/4/14.

65. Rainie, L. 2013. Cellphone ownership hits 91% of adults. *Pew Research Center.* http://www.pewresearch. org/fact-tank/2013/06/06/cell-phone-ownership-hits-91-of-adults. Accessed 5/4/14.

66. Ericsson. 2014. Ericsson Mobility Report. http://www.ericsson.com/ericsson-mobility-report. Accessed 5/4/14.

67. Nielsen. 2013. Mobile majority: U.S. smartphone ownership tops 60%. http://www.nielsen.com/us/en/ newswire /2013/mobile-majority—u-s—smartphone-ownership-tops-60-.html. Accessed 4/5/14.

68. Canadian Press. 2014. Canadian smartphone users spend lots of time staring at screens: Poll. *Global News.* http://globalnews.ca/news/1067393/canadian-smart-phone-users-spend-lots-of-time-staring-at-screens-poll. Accessed 4/5/14.

69. Schüz, J., et al. 2006. Cellular telephone use and cancer risk: Update of a nation-wide Danish cohort. *Journal of the National Cancer Institute* 98(23): 1707–13.

70. Serrano, T. 2013. Israeli study shows cellphone radiation and thyroid cancer link. http://blog.cellphone-health.com/2013/03/israeli-study-shows-cell-phone-radiation-thyroid-cancer-link.html. Accessed 4/5/14.

71. Hamzany et al. 2013. Is human saliva an indicator of the adverse health effects of using mobile phones? *Antioxidants and Redox Signaling* 18(6): 622–27.

72. National Cancer Institute. Surveillance, Epidemiology, and End Results Program: Stats fact sheet—thyroid cancer. http://seer.cancer.gov/statfacts/html/ thyro.html. Accessed 4/4/14.

73. Milham, S. 2009. Most cancer in firefighters is due to radio-frequency radiation exposure not inhaled carcinogens. *Medical Hypotheses* 73(5): 788–89.

74. Mortavazi et al. 2009. Alterations in TSH and thyroid hormones following mobile phone use. *Oman Medical Journal* 24(4): 274–78.

75. Matavulj et al. 1999. Electromagnetic field effects on the morphology of rat thyroid gland. *Electricity and Magnetism in Biology and Medicine* 489–92.

76. Hillert et al. 2008. The effects of 884 MHz GSM wireless communication signals on headache and other symptoms: An experimental provocation study. *Bioelectromagnetics* 29(3): 185–96.

77. Thomée et al. 2011. Mobile phone use and stress, sleep disturbances, and symptoms of depression among young adults: A prospective cohort study. *BMC Public Health* 11: 66.

78. Lajunen et al. 2007. Are computer and cellphone use associated with body mass index and overweight? A population study among twin adolescents. *BMC Public Health* 7: 24.

79. Gittleman, A.L. 2010. *Zapped: Why Your Cell Phone Shouldn't Be Your Alarm Clock and 1,268 Ways to Outsmart the Hazards of Electronic Pollution.* New York: HarperCollins.

80. Lepp et al. 2013. The relationship between cellphone use, physical and sedentary activity, and cardiorespiratory fitness in a sample of U.S. college students. *International Journal of Behavioral Nutrition and Physical Activity* 10: 79.

81. Wright, V. 2014. The benefits of a morning walk for a good night's sleep (video). http://www.huffingtonpost.com/2014/01/04/sleep-better-morning-walk_n_4519660.html. Accessed 3/5/14.

82. Davis, J.L. Lose weight with morning exercise. WebMD Feature. http://www.webmd.com/fitness-exercise/features/lose-weight-with-morning-exercise. Accessed 3/5/14.

83. Washington State University Nutrition Education. 2013. Eat together, eat better leader's guide. http://nutrition.wsu.edu/ETEB/pdf/LeadersGuide/ETEBLeader-Guide.pdf. Accessed 3/4/14.

84. Hammons, A.J., and Fiese, B.H. 2011. Is frequency of shared family meals related to the nutritional health of children and adolescents? *Pediatrics* 127(6): e1565–74.

85. CASA. 2007. The importance of family dinners. http://www.casacolumbia.org/addiction-research/reports/importance-of-family-dinners-2007. Accessed 5/6/14.

86. Daubenmier et al. 2011. Mindfulness intervention for stress eating to reduce cortisol and abdominal fat among overweight and obese women: An exploratory randomized controlled study. *Journal of Obesity* 2011: 651936.

87. Lenze et al. 2014. Mindfulness-based stress reduction for older adults with worry symptoms and co-occurring cognitive dysfunction. *International Journal of Geriatric Psychiatry* [Epub ahead of print].

88. Meadows et al. 2014. Mindfulness-based cognitive therapy for recurrent depression: A translational research study with 2-year follow-up. *Australian and New Zealand Journal of Psychiatry* [Epub ahead of print].

89. Regehr et al. 2013. Interventions to reduce stress in university students: A review and meta-analysis. *Journal of Affective Disorders* 148(1): 1–11.

90. Jacobs et al. 2013. Self-reported mindfulness and cortisol during a Shamatha meditation retreat. *Health Psychology* 32(10): 1104–09.

91. Ferrarelli et al. 2013. Experienced mindfulness meditators exhibit higher parietal-occipital EEG gamma activity during NREM sleep. *PLoS One* 8(8): e73417.

92. Carlson et al. 2007. One year pre-post intervention follow-up of psychological, immune, endocrine and blood pressure outcomes of mindfulness-based stress reduction (MBSR) in breast and prostate cancer outpatients. *Brain, Behavior, and Immunity* 21(8): 1038–49.

93. Witek-Janusek et al. 2008. Effect of mindfulness-based stress reduction on immune function, quality of life and coping in women newly diagnosed with early stage breast cancer. *Brain, Behavior, and Immunity* 22(6): 969–81.

94. Daubenmier et al. 2011. Mindfulness intervention for stress eating to reduce cortisol and abdominal fat among overweight and obese women: an exploratory randomized controlled study. *Journal of Obesity* 2011(2011): 651936.

95. Mantzios, M., and Giannou, K. 2014. Group vs. single mindfulness meditation: Exploring avoidance, impulsivity, and weight management in two separate mindfulness meditation settings. *Applied Psychology Health Well-Being* [Epub ahead of print].

96. Courbasson et al. 2011. Mindfulness-action based cognitive behavioral therapy for concurrent binge eating disorder and substance use disorders. *Eating Disorders* 19(1): 17–33.

97. Brown et al. 1995. Chronic psychological effects of exercise and exercise plus cognitive strategies. *Medicine and Science in Sports and Exercise* 27(5): 765–75.

CHAPTER 7: SAY YES TO SUCCESS

1. Buman et al. 2011. Moderators and mediators of exercise-induced objective sleep improvements in midlife and older adults with sleep complaints. *Health Psychology* 30(5): 579–87.

2. Foster-Schubert et al. 2012. Effect of diet and exercise, alone or combined, on weight and body composition in overweight-to-obese postmenopausal women. *Obesity* (Silver Spring) 20(8): 1628–38.

3. Bast, E.S., and Berry, E.M. 2014. Laugh away the fat? Therapeutic humor in the control of stress-induced emotional eating. *Rambam Maimonides Medical Journal* 5(1): e0007.

4. Berk et al. 1989. Neuroendocrine and stress hormone changes during mirthful laughter. *American Journal of the Medical Sciences* 298: 390–96.

5. Buchowski et al. 2007. Energy expenditure of genuine laughter. *International Journal of Obesity* 31(1): 131–7.

6. Hollis et al. 2008. Weight loss during the intensive intervention phase of the weight-loss maintenance trial. *American Journal of Preventative Medicine* 35(2): 118–26.

7. Elfhag, K., and Rossner, S. 2005. Who succeeds in maintaining weight loss? A conceptual review of factors associated with weight loss maintenance and weight regain. *Obesity Reviews* 6(1): 67-85.

8. Gorin, A., et al. 2005. Involving support partners in obesity treatment. *Journal of Consulting and Clinical Psychology* 73(2): 341–43.

9. Astrup, A., and Rossner, S. 2000. Lessons from obesity management programmes: Greater initial weight loss improves long-term maintenance. *Obesity Reviews* 1(1): 17–19.

10. Nackers, L.M., Ross, K.M., and Perri, M.G. 2010. The association between rate of initial weight loss and long-term success in obesity treatment: Does slow and steady win the race? *International Journal of Behavioral Medicine* 17(3): 161–67.

CHAPTER 8: MY 5 FOR LIFE

1. Wing, R.R., and Phelan, S. 2005 Long-term weight loss maintenance. *American Journal of Clinical Nutrition* 82(1): 222S–5S.

2. Gorin et al. 2004. Promoting long-term weight control: Does dieting consistency matter? *International Journal of Obesity and Related Metabolism Disorders* 28(2): 278–81.

3. http://www.realage.com.

4. Metcalfe et al. 2012. Towards the minimal amount of exercise for improving metabolic health: Beneficial effects of reduced-exertion high-intensity interval training. *European Journal of Applied Physiology* 112(7): 2767–75.

5. Burgomaster et al. 2008. Similar metabolic adaptations during exercise after low volume sprint interval and traditional endurance training in humans. *Journal of Physiology* 586(1): 151–60.

6. Fan et al. 2013. Moderate to vigorous physical activity and weight outcomes: Does every minute count? *American Journal of Health Promotion* 28(1): 41–49.

7. Macpherson et al. 2011. Run sprint interval training improves aerobic performance but not maximal cardiac output. *Medicine and Science in Sports and Exercise* 43(1): 115–22.

8. Terada et al. 2004. Effect of high-intensity intermittent swimming training on fatty acid oxidation enzyme activity in rat skeletal muscle. *Japanese Journal of Physiology* 54(1): 47–52.

9. Dolan et al. 2006. "Take the stairs instead of the escalator": Effect of environmental prompts on community stair use and implications for a national "Small Steps" campaign. *Obesity Review* 7(1): 25–32.

10. Harvard Medical School. 2009. Walking: Your steps to health. http://www.health.harvard.edu/newsletters/Harvard_Mens_Health_Watch/2009/August/Walking-Your-steps-to-health.

11. Benn et al. 1996. Circulatory responses to weight lifting, walking, and stair climbing in older males. *Journal of the American Geriatrics Society* 44(2): 121–25.

CHAPTER 9: WHY YOU'LL NEVER REGAIN THE POUNDS

1. Lewis, M., Obama's Way. *Vanity Fair.* http://www.vanityfair.com/politics/2012/10/michael-lewis-profile-barack-obama. Accessed 5/11/14.

2. Lally, P. et al., "How are habits formed: Modelling habit formation in the real world." *European Journal of Social Psychology* 40(6): 998–1009.

3. Muraven, M., and Baumeister, R.F. 2000. Self-regulation and depletion of limited resources: Does self-control resemble a muscle? *Psychological Bulletin* 126(2): 247–59.

4. Oaten, M., and Cheng, K. 2006. Longitudinal gains in self-regulation from regular physical exercise. *British Journal of Health and Psychology* 11(Pt 4): 717–33.

5. Neal, D.T., et al. 2011. How do habits guide behavior? Perceived and actual triggers of habits in daily life. *Journal of Experimental Social Psychology* 48(2): 492–98.

6. Danner, U.N., et al. 2008. Habit vs. intention in the prediction of future behavior: The role of frequency, context stability and mental accessibility of past behavior. *British Journal of Social Psychology* 47: 245–65.

7. NPR. 2012. Habits: How they form and how to break them (transcript). http://www.npr.org/2012/03/05/147192599/habits-how-they-form-and-how-to-break-them. Accessed 5/11/14.

8. Vohs, K., et al. 2008. Making choices impairs subsequent self-control: A limited-resource account of decision making, self-regulation, and active initiative. *Journal of Personality and Social Psychology* 94(5): 882–98.

9. McGuire, M.T., et al. 1999. Behavioral strategies of individuals who have maintained long-term weight losses. *Obesity Research* 7(4): 334–41.

10. Reyes, N.R., et al. 2012. Similarities and differences between weight loss maintainers and regainers: A qualitative analysis. *Journal of the Academy of Nutrition and Dietetics* 112(4): 499–505.

11. Elfhag, K., and Rössner, S. 2005. Who succeeds in maintaining weight loss? A conceptual review of factors associated with weight loss maintenance and weight regain. *Obesity Review* 6(1): 67–85.

12. Kong, A. 2012. Adoption of diet-related self-monitoring behaviors varies by race/ethnicity, education, and baseline binge eating score among overweight-to-obese postmenopausal women in a 12-month dietary weight loss intervention. *Nutrition Research* 32(4): 260–65.

INDEX

Boldface page references indicate illustrations. <u>Underscored</u> references indicate tables or boxed text.

A

Activity monitors, 69–71, <u>73</u>
Add Variety workout, 157–58, 224–31
Aerobic or cardiovascular exercise. *See also* Walking
    climbing stairs, 153–54, <u>153</u>
    forms of, <u>57</u>
    health benefits of, <u>53</u>
    increasing, 149–55, <u>158</u>
    moderate and consistent, 73–74
    other activities, <u>155</u>
    overexercising, 65–66, <u>65</u>
    resistance exercise vs., <u>34</u>
    sprints, 151–53
Almonds, as weight loss aid, <u>22</u>
Ambien, 91
Amish people, 51
Appetite. *See also* Satiety
    hormones affecting, 81–82
    overexercising and, 65, <u>65</u>, <u>73</u>
Apples
    Apple, Peach, and Spinach Smoothie, 180
    PB and Grape Smoothie, 179
Artichokes
    Artichoke, Mushroom, and Smoked Salmon Scramble, 181
Arugula
    Cumin-Roasted Sweet Potato, Quinoa, and Black Bean Salad, 191
    White Bean, Caramelized Onion, and Wilted Arugula Toast, 187
Asparagus
    Spring Green Sauté with Farro, 205
Avocado
    Chocolate-Avocado Mousse with Raspberries, 212
    eating with meat, <u>22</u>
    Skinny Guacamole, 211
    South-of-the-Border Omelet, 183
    Spinach Omelet with Feta and Avocado, 182
    Tropical Green Smoothie, 178

B

Balance, exercise improving, 35
Ball Hamstring Curl, 228, **228**
Bananas
    PB and Grape Smoothie, 179
    Tropical Green Smoothie, 178
Barley
    Turkey, Barley, and Chard Soup, 199
Beans and legumes
    bloating or gas from, 11
    Creamy White Bean and Kale Soup, 201
    Cumin-Roasted Sweet Potato, Quinoa, and Black Bean Salad, 191
    guidelines for, 17–18
    Kale Salad with Toasted Chickpeas and Lemon-Tahini Dressing, 193
    Mediterranean Lemon-Chicken Soup, 200
    as protein source, 11
    Red Lentil Puree, 209
    Shrimp and Black Bean Stir-Fry, 202
    South-of-the-Border Omelet, 183
    White Bean, Caramelized Onion, and Wilted Arugula Toast, 187
Bedding, <u>89</u>
Bedroom environment, 88, <u>92</u>, <u>93</u>
Beef. *See* Meat
Behavior, habits vs., 162, <u>172</u>
Bell pepper
    Bell Pepper and Turkey Roll-Ups, 208
Berries
    Berry-Muesli Yogurt Parfait, 213
    Blueberry-Pomegranate Slushie, 177

Beverages, 23
Blood sugar, exercise and, 33–34
Blueberries. *See* Berries
Body mass index (BMI), 80–81, 84, 112–13
Bone density, exercise and, 35
Brain, 67–68, 86–87
Bread, guidelines for, <u>14</u>
Breakfast, 11, <u>12</u>, <u>24</u>, 128
Breathing during exercise, <u>39</u>

C

Calories
  burned by walking, 60–61
  burning at rest, 36–37, 38
  daily amount of, 5
  portion control for, 5, 123–24
  protein vs. carb, 5
  satiety and, 5–6
  weight loss and burning of, 38
Carbohydrates. *See also* Fruit; Vegetables
  benefits of fibrous, 14
  calories in protein vs., 5
  choosing ones with fiber, 14
  guidelines for, <u>24</u>
  importance of, 13
  low-carb diets, 13–14
  non-starchy, 15
Cardio machines, <u>155</u>
Cardiovascular exercise. *See* Aerobic or
    cardiovascular exercise
Cellphones. *See* Electronic devices
Chard
  Turkey, Barley, and Chard Soup, 199
Cheese. *See also* Dairy
  Grilled Cheese, Pear, and Turkey Sandwich, 188
  Italian Frittata with Zucchini, Leeks, and
    Parmesan, 185
  Salmon and Goat Cheese Melt, 186
  Spinach Omelet with Feta and Avocado, 182
Chicken. *See* Poultry
Chocolate
  Chocolate-Avocado Mousse with Raspberries,
    212
Chronic movement. *See also* Walking
  activity monitors for, 69–71, <u>73</u>
  being less efficient, 55–57, <u>56</u>
  exercise vs., 49–50, 72
  fitting into life, 55, 56–58, <u>56</u>
  health benefits of, <u>53</u>
  inhibitors of, <u>57</u>
  more steps per day, 149–50
  as non-exercise activity thermogenesis, 25,
    52–53

statistics, 55
technology and decline in, 52
10,000 steps a day, 53–55, 69, 71, 73, 149–50
tips for increasing, <u>71</u>
traditional vs. modern, 50–51
underrated, 25–26, 49
Climbing stairs, 153–54, <u>153</u>
Clock, body's, 77, 82–83, 85, <u>97</u>
Computers. *See* Electronic devices
Condiments, recommended, 13
Continuous positive airway pressure (CPAP)
    devices, 91
Corn
  Charred Corn and Cumin Chicken Wrap, 189
  Manhattan-Style Chicken-Corn Chowder,
    198
Cortisol, 83, <u>97</u>

D

Dairy. *See also* Cheese; Yogurt
  guidelines for, 9
  shopping for, 126
  smoothies, 176–80
Dancing, <u>155</u>
Day 6 and beyond. *See also* Habits
  aerobic activity, 149–55
  modifications to the plan, 145
  resistance exercise, 156–59
  treating yourself, 148–49
  variety in diet, 147–48, <u>148</u>
  weighing yourself, 145–46, <u>158</u>
  weight loss and, 147, 170–71
Decision-making stress, 168–70
Depression, walking and, 68
Diet. *See* My 5 eating plan
Dinner recommendations, 129
Drinks, 23
Drugs for sleep, avoiding, 91–94
Dumbbell Hammer Biceps Curl, 238, **238**
Dumbbell Lateral Raise, 229, **229**
Dumbbells, purchasing, 40–41
Dumbbell Single-Arm Triceps Kickback, 227, **227**

E

Earplugs, 90
Eggplant
  Steak and Ratatouille Stir-Fry, 206
Eggs
  Lite French Toast, 207
  as protein source, 11
  scrambles, 181–85
  whites vs. yolks, 11

Electronic devices
app for Internet blocking, <u>109</u>
avoiding before bed, 86, 96
blue light from, 85, 108, <u>108</u>, <u>118</u>
cellphone radiation, 109, 110–12, <u>111</u>
cellphone safety, <u>110</u>
cellphones and weight, 112–13
changing trends, <u>102</u>
eating changed by, 101–2
electro-pollution from, <u>112</u>
hours per day spent with, 98–99
ills with computer use, 103–4
information push, <u>105</u>
kids' use of, <u>107</u>
lockout device for TV, 102
media multitasking, 106–7
men vs. women and, 102
sitting due to, 114, <u>118</u>
sleep deprivation and, 78, 79, 85, 108, 111–12
social media and emotional health, 105–6
stress-reduction at work, 104–5
text neck due to, 113–14
thyroid health and, 110–11, <u>111</u>, <u>118</u>
TV's impact, 100, <u>100</u>, 103
unplugging, 99, 114–15, 145
using time freed from, 115–17
weight gain and, 99–100, <u>100</u>, 101–2, <u>118</u>
Emotional health, social media and, 105–6
Exercise. See Aerobic or cardiovascular exercise;
    Chronic movement; Resistance exercise

F
Farro
Spring Green Sauté with Farro, 205
Fats
author's favorites, <u>22</u>
benefits of eating, <u>22</u>
guidelines for, <u>21</u>, 22–23
importance of, 21–22, <u>24</u>
shopping for, 126
table summarizing, <u>21</u>
Fiber
benefits of eating, 19–20
choosing carbs with, 14
daily amount of, 19
fruits high in, <u>17</u>
in legumes, 11
soluble and insoluble, <u>20</u>
Fibrous carbohydrates. See Carbohydrates
Fish. See Seafood
Fitness level assessment, 46–47
Free meals, 148–49, <u>158</u>
Frequent urination, <u>87</u>

Fruit. See also specific kinds
guidelines for, 16
high fiber, <u>17</u>
importance of, 15
shopping for, 126
smoothies, 176–80

G
Game. See Meat
Get Started workout, 216–23
Ghrelin, 81–82, <u>97</u>
Glycemic index (GI), <u>19</u>
Goal setting, <u>139</u>
Golf, <u>57</u>, 116
Grains, 17, <u>18</u>, 126
Grapes
PB and Grape Smoothie, 179
Grazing, 4, 5
Greek yogurt. See Yogurt
Green beans
Salad Niçoise, 196

H
Habits
bad, 161–62
behavior vs., 162, <u>172</u>
goal needed to form, 164–65
habit loop, 165–67, <u>172</u>
mindfulness and, 168, <u>172</u>
preventing, 165–67, <u>166</u>
repetition and, 167–68
time required to form, 163
tips for developing, <u>167</u>, <u>169</u>
usefulness of, 160–61, <u>172</u>
willpower and, 163–64
Halcion, 91, 92
Hash
Sweet Potato Hash with Turkey Sausage, 184
Hiking, <u>155</u>
Hip Thrust, 226, **226**, 234
Hormones
cellphones and, 110–11
insulin, 14–15, 36, 38, 39
released by exercise, 35
sleep and, 81–83, <u>97</u>

I
Immune system, 66, 79
Inactivity, ills due to, <u>60</u>, 78
Injury risk, walking and, 69
Inline skating, <u>155</u>

Insoluble fiber, 20
Insomnia, 79–80
Insulin, 14–15, 36
Insulin resistance, 38, 39
Internet. *See* Electronic devices

J

Jerky for snacks, 124
Jogging, 62, 64, 68, 151
Journal keeping, 139–40

K

Kale
    Creamy White Bean and Kale Soup, 201
    Kale Salad with Toasted Chickpeas and
        Lemon-Tahini Dressing, 193

L

Laughter, 134
Leading by example, 141, 143
Leeks
    Italian Frittata with Zucchini, Leeks, and
        Parmesan, 185
    Mediterranean Lemon-Chicken Soup, 200
Legumes. *See* Beans and legumes
Lentils. *See* Beans and legumes
Leptin, 81, 97
Lettuce
    Chopped Chicken and Pepperoni Salad on
        Mixed Greens, 194–95
    Salad Niçoise, 196
Life expectancy, TV and, 103
Light, sleep and, 78, 84–86
Low-carb diets, 13–14
Lunch recommendations, 129
Lunesta, 91
Lying Dumbbell Triceps Extension, 219, **219**,
    234, **234**
Lying Trunk Twist, 240, **240**

M

Macronutrients, 6. *See also* Carbohydrates; Fats;
    Protein
Mattresses, 92
Meal plans, 126–30
Meat. *See also* Poultry
    as protein source, 10
    Steak and Ratatouille Stir-Fry, 206
Media multitasking, 106–7
Meditation, 116, 117–18, 168, 172

Melatonin, 82–83, 97
Memory, improved by exercise, 68
Metabolism
    basal (resting), defined, 67
    benefits of raising, 35, 73
    calorie burning and, 37
    exercise type and, 32–33
    overexercising and, 64
    workout after-burn, 36
Mindfulness, 117–18, 168, 172
Motivation, 62, 63, 142–43
Movement. *See* Chronic movement
Muscles
    built by exercise, 34–35, 38
    bulk concerns, 26–27, 44–45
    calories burned at rest by, 36–37
    names of, 45
    targeting key groups, 43–44
    working opposing, 46
Mushrooms
    Artichoke, Mushroom, and Smoked Salmon
        Scramble, 181
    Korean Chicken Stir-Fry, 204
My 5 eating plan
    adding variety, 147–48, 148, 158
    benefits of grazing, 5
    frequency for eating, 3–4, 24
    guidelines for, 3
    meal plans, 126–30
    no-time-to-cook meals, 127, 127
    not sufficient by itself, 2
    portion control, 123–24
    reasons it's easy, 3
    in restaurants, 120–22, 121
    shopping for, 125–26
    simple formula for, 2
    sleep and, 84
    treating yourself, 148–49, 158
    types of meals in, 123
My 5 Plan. *See also* Day 6 and beyond
    fitting into life, 137–38, 143
    gestalt of, 133–35, 143
    initial weight loss in, 141–42
    journal keeping, 139–40
    motivation in, 142–43
    prioritizing for, 138, 139
    questions to ask, 131–33, 135, 143, 144, 158
    turning around mishaps, 135–37
    using your time well, 139
    willpower and, 140–41
My 5 workouts
    Add Variety, 157–58, 224–31
    calories burned between, 37
    Get Started, 216–23

program summary, 216, <u>216</u>
Take It Up a Notch, 159, 232–42

N

Nightlights, 85, 86
No, saying, <u>139</u>
Noise, sleep deprivation and, 78
Non-exercise activity thermogenesis (NEAT), 25, 52–53. *See also* Chronic movement
No-time-to-cook meals, 127, <u>127</u>

O

Oats, <u>18</u>
Obesity
    Amish vs. other Americans, 51
    car use vs. walking and, 58–59
    global increase in, 104
    sitting and, 55
    TV watching and, 101–2
Olive oil, <u>22</u>
Omelets. *See* Scrambles
Onions
    White Bean, Caramelized Onion, and Wilted Arugula Toast, 187

P

Pace of walking, 62–63, 150
Peaches
    Apple, Peach, and Spinach Smoothie, 180
    Green Ginger-Peach Smoothie, 176
Pears
    Grilled Cheese, Pear, and Turkey Sandwich, 188
    Pear Crumble with Greek Yogurt, 210
Peas
    Skinny Guacamole, 211
    Spring Green Sauté with Farro, 205
Pedometers, 69–71, <u>73</u>
Pike Plank, 233, **233**
Pillows, <u>93</u>
Pomegranate
    Blueberry-Pomegranate Slushie, 177
Pork. *See* Meat
Portion control, 5, 123–24
Potatoes
    Manhattan-Style Chicken-Corn Chowder, 198
    nutrition in, <u>16</u>
Poultry
    Bell Pepper and Turkey Roll-Ups, 208
    Charred Corn and Cumin Chicken Wrap, 189

Chopped Chicken and Pepperoni Salad on Mixed Greens, 194–95
    Curried Chicken and Baby Spinach Salad, 190
    Green Split Pea Soup, 197
    Grilled Cheese, Pear, and Turkey Sandwich, 188
    Korean Chicken Stir-Fry, 204
    Manhattan-Style Chicken-Corn Chowder, 198
    Mediterranean Lemon-Chicken Soup, 200
    as protein source, 9
    Sweet Potato Hash with Turkey Sausage, 184
    Turkey, Barley, and Chard Soup, 199
Protein
    benefits of eating, 7
    at breakfast, 11, <u>12</u>, <u>24</u>
    calories in carbs vs., 5
    importance of, 7, <u>24</u>
    not stored by the body, 6–7
    shopping for, 125–26
    sources of, 8–12
Protein powder, 12. *See also* Smoothies
Pumpkin seeds, <u>22</u>
Pushup, 240, 242, **242**

Q

Questions to ask yourself, 131–33, 135, <u>143</u>, 144, <u>158</u>
Quiet time, 116–17
Quinoa
    about, <u>18</u>
    Cumin-Roasted Sweet Potato, Quinoa, and Black Bean Salad, 191
    Saffron Shrimp Paella, 203

R

Rapid eye movement (REM) sleep, <u>90</u>
Raspberries. *See* Berries
Recipes, 173–213
    index by types, 174–75
    salads, 190–96
    sandwiches, 186–89
    scrambles, 181–85
    smoothies, 176–80
    snacks, 207–13
    soups, 197–201
    stir-fries and skillet dishes, 202–6
Resistance exercise, 25–48
    adding variety, 156–58, <u>156</u>
    Add Variety workout, 157–58, 224–31
    advanced level tips, <u>157</u>
    assessing fitness level for, 46–47

Resistance exercise (*cont.*)
  avoiding plateaus, 42
  benefits of, 34–40, <u>48</u>
  breathing during, <u>39</u>
  cardiovascular exercise vs., <u>34</u>
  concerns about, 26–27, 30, 44–45
  cooldown for, 47
  Day 6 and beyond, 156–59
  described, 26, <u>48</u>
  5-day tryout for, 30–31
  5-minute approach to, 27, 30, 42–43, 45–46, <u>48</u>
  Get Started workout, 216–23
  increasing, 156–59
  making it a habit, 41–42
  muscle group targeting, 43–44
  order of exercises, 45–46
  preconceived ideas about, 27
  principles of My 5 Plan, 29
  program summary, 216, <u>216</u>
  reasons why My 5 is easy, <u>36</u>
  repetitions, defined, <u>43</u>
  research supporting, 31–34
  revolutionary approach to, 27
  sets, defined, <u>43</u>
  stumbling blocks to, 28
  Take It Up a Notch workout, 159, 232–42
  types of, 26
  warmup for, 47
  weights for, 40–41
  working opposing muscles, <u>46</u>
Restaurants, ordering in, 120–22, <u>121</u>
Restoril, 91, 92
Reverse Fly, 230, **230**
Reverse Lunge, 217, **217**, 233
Running
  adding to your regimen, 151
  sprints, 151–53
  walking vs., 62, <u>64</u>, <u>68</u>
Rye, <u>18</u>

S

Safety when walking, <u>72</u>
Salads, 190–96
  Chopped Chicken and Pepperoni Salad on
    Mixed Greens, 194–95
  Cumin-Roasted Sweet Potato, Quinoa, and
    Black Bean Salad, 191
  Curried Chicken and Baby Spinach Salad, 190
  Kale Salad with Toasted Chickpeas and
    Lemon-Tahini Dressing, 193
  Salad Niçoise, 196
  Spicy, Crunchy Wheat Berry Salad, 192

Sandwiches, 186–89
  Charred Corn and Cumin Chicken Wrap, 189
  Grilled Cheese, Pear, and Turkey Sandwich,
    188
  Salmon and Goat Cheese Melt, 186
  White Bean, Caramelized Onion, and Wilted
    Arugula Toast, 187
Satiety. *See also* Appetite
  food types and, 5–6
  holy trinity of, 122
  olive oil inducing, <u>22</u>
Sauces, recommended, 13
Scheduling, <u>139</u>
Scrambles, 181–85
  Artichoke, Mushroom, and Smoked Salmon
    Scramble, 181
  Italian Frittata with Zucchini, Leeks, and
    Parmesan, 185
  South-of-the-Border Omelet, 183
  Spinach Omelet with Feta and Avocado, 182
  Sweet Potato Hash with Turkey Sausage, 184
Seafood
  Artichoke, Mushroom, and Smoked Salmon
    Scramble, 181
  good choices for, <u>8</u>
  HDL raised by salmon, <u>22</u>
  as protein source, 8
  Saffron Shrimp Paella, 203
  Salad Niçoise, 196
  Salmon and Goat Cheese Melt, 186
  Shrimp and Black Bean Stir-Fry, 202
Seated Trunk Twist, 235, **235**
Seeds, <u>20</u>
Serotonin, sleep and, 83
Shoes, walking, <u>70</u>
Shopping for food, 125–26
Shrimp. *See* Seafood
Side Plank, 231, **231**
Single-Arm Dumbbell Row, 222, **222**, 237, **237**
Single-Leg Tap Squat, 225, **225**
Sitting
  electronic devices and, 114, <u>118</u>
  ills due to, <u>60</u>
  obesity and, 55
  postural issues with, 114
Skating, <u>155</u>
Skillet dishes. *See* Stir-fries and skillet dishes
Skyr (Icelandic yogurt), <u>10</u>
Sleep, 75–97
  author's need for, 75
  benefits of enough, 87–88
  blue light from screens and, 108, <u>118</u>
  cellphones and, 111–12

Day 6 and beyond, 145
daytime strategies aiding, 95
devices aiding, 90–91
diet and, 84
drugs for, avoiding, 91–94
factors affecting, 77–78
frequent urination and, 87
hormones and, 81–83, 97
ills due to lack of, 79, 97
importance of, 77
insomnia, 79–80
light and, 84–86
mattress for, 92
pillow for, 93
power naps, 76
preparing for, 86, 88–90, 97, 115
prevalence of lack, 76
REM, 90
shift in thinking about, 75–76
sleepmate issues, 94
after waking, 96
weight and, 80–81, 85, 86–87
Sleep apnea, 85
Sleeping pills, avoiding, 91–94
Sleep masks, 90
Sleep monitors, 90–91
Slim appearance, creating, 39–40
Smoothies, 176–80
    Apple, Peach, and Spinach Smoothie,
        180
    Blueberry-Pomegranate Slushie, 177
    Green Ginger-Peach Smoothie, 176
    PB and Grape Smoothie, 179
    Tropical Green Smoothie, 178
Snacks, 207–13
    Bell Pepper and Turkey Roll-Ups, 208
    Berry-Muesli Yogurt Parfait, 213
    calories per snack, 5
    Chocolate-Avocado Mousse with Raspberries,
        212
    ingredients in, 122
    jerky for, 124
    Lite French Toast, 207
    Pear Crumble with Greek Yogurt, 210
    portions in, 124
    Red Lentil Puree, 209
    shopping for, 126
    Skinny Guacamole, 211
    suggestions, 124–25
Social media, emotional health and, 105–6
Soluble fiber, 20
Sonata, 91
Sound-masking devices, 90

Soups, 197–201
    Creamy White Bean and Kale Soup, 201
    Green Split Pea Soup, 197
    Manhattan-Style Chicken-Corn Chowder,
        198
    Mediterranean Lemon-Chicken Soup, 200
    Turkey, Barley, and Chard Soup, 199
Spinach
    Apple, Peach, and Spinach Smoothie, 180
    Chopped Chicken and Pepperoni Salad on
        Mixed Greens, 194–95
    Curried Chicken and Baby Spinach Salad, 190
    Green Ginger-Peach Smoothie, 176
    Korean Chicken Stir-Fry, 204
    Spicy, Crunchy Wheat Berry Salad, 192
    Spinach Omelet with Feta and Avocado, 182
Split peas
    Green Split Pea Soup, 197
Sports, 155
Sprints, 151–53
Stair walking, 153–54, 153
Standing Dumbbell Curl Press, 221, 221
Standing Dumbbell Shoulder Press, 235, 236,
    236
Standing Dumbbell Side Bend, 223, 223, 234,
    234
Starchy vegetables, 16
Stiff-Leg Dumbbell Deadlift, 220, 220, 234
Stir-fries and skillet dishes, 202–6
    Korean Chicken Stir-Fry, 204
    Saffron Shrimp Paella, 203
    Shrimp and Black Bean Stir-Fry, 202
    Spring Green Sauté with Farro, 205
    Steak and Ratatouille Stir-Fry, 206
Strength training. See Resistance exercise
Stress
    of decision making, 168–70
    reducing, 69, 117–18
    serotonin reduced by, 83
    sleep deprivation and, 78, 83
Sumo Squat, 240, 241, 241
Sunlight, 84
Superman, 218, 218, 237
Sweet potatoes
    Cumin-Roasted Sweet Potato, Quinoa, and
        Black Bean Salad, 191
    Sweet Potato Hash with Turkey Sausage, 184
Swimming, 155

T

Tablets. See Electronic devices
Take It Up a Notch workout, 159, 232–42

Technology, 52. *See also* Electronic devices
Television. *See* Electronic devices
Temperature for sleeping, 89
10,000 steps a day, 53–55, 69, 71, 73, 149–50. *See also* Chronic movement
Text neck, avoiding, 113–14
Thyroid health, cellphone radiation and, 110–11, 111, 118
Treating yourself, 148–49, 158
Turkey. *See* Poultry

U

Urination, frequent, 87

V

Vegetables. *See also specific kinds*
  guidelines for, 15–16
  importance of, 15
  shopping for, 126
  starchy, 16
Video games. *See* Electronic devices

W

Walking
  all at once vs. throughout the day, 61–62
  amount needed, 63–64
  benefits of, 67–69, 73
  brain stimulated by, 67–68
  calories burned by, 60–61
  depression reduced by, 68
  fitting into life, 55, 56–58, 56
  on an incline, 154–55
  injury risk reduced by, 69
  motivators for, 62, 63
  pace of, 62–63, 150
  running or jogging vs., 62, 64, 68
  safety guidelines, 72
  shoes for, 70
  on stairs, 153–54, 153
  statistics, 55
  stress reduced by, 69
  in 10 healthiest countries vs. U.S., 59–60
  tips for, 54, 55, 62
  weight gain avoided by, 61

Warmup for exercise, 47
Water, daily amount of, 23
Weighing yourself, 145–46, 158
Weight gain
  avoiding with exercise, 39, 61
  electronic devices and, 99–100, 100, 101–2, 118
  sleep and, 80, 86–87
  sleep apnea and, 85
Weight loss
  almonds aiding, 22
  calorie burning reduced by, 38
  checking the scale for, 145–46
  continuing to lose weight, 147
  fiber's benefits for, 19–20
  initial rapid, 141–42
  keeping it off, 170–71
  laughter aiding, 134
  sleep and, 80–81
Weights, purchasing, 40–41
Weight training. *See* Resistance exercise
Wheat berries
  about, 18
  Spicy, Crunchy Wheat Berry Salad, 192
Whole grains, 17, 18, 126
Wild rice, 18
Willpower, not needed, 140–41
Work, sleep deprivation and, 77
Workouts. *See* My 5 workouts
Wraps. *See* Sandwiches

Y

Yogurt. *See also* Dairy
  Berry-Muesli Yogurt Parfait, 213
  Curried Chicken and Baby Spinach Salad, 190
  Greek vs. regular, 10
  Icelandic-style skyr, 10
  Pear Crumble with Greek Yogurt, 210

Z

Zucchini
  Italian Frittata with Zucchini, Leeks, and Parmesan, 185
  Steak and Ratatouille Stir-Fry, 206